The 7 ESSENTIAL HAIRCUTS *for* WOMEN

By NIKKI MORGAN ALLEN

Illustrated by MELANIE LA MAY
and NIKKI MORGAN ALLEN
Color by BOB ALLEN

INTRODUCTION

Welcome to The 7 ESSENTIAL HAIRCUTS for WOMEN!

This book Illustrates The Oval Haircut, The One Length Haircut, The A-Line Haircut, The Bob Haircut, The Inverted Bob Haircut, The Bi-Level Haircut and The Pixie Haircut.

Each of these haircuts have lots of variations, so I am sure you will find the haircut you are looking for!

All the haircuts are shown in a large image with a front view, side view and back view.

Each haircut is followed by a page, or two, of 4 smaller images with different options for that haircut.

Every great haircut starts with a great consultation and The 7 ESSENTIAL HAIRCUTS for WOMEN bridges the gap between hairstylist and client for a picture-perfect haircut every time!

CONTENTS

FACE SHAPE

A great haircut is tailored to our facial bone structure. Our faces come in many different shapes. Oval, Square, Rectangle, Heart, Oblong, Round, Triangle, Diamond and everything in between.

Hairstylists are often asked which haircut is best for my face shape?

The best answer is we want to highlight our best features. And downplay our problem areas.

Most haircuts can be customized to work with most face shapes.

For example, if your face shape is narrow, you might want to add layers to your haircut to give the illusion of width and volume. For a wider face shape, you might want to try a longer length haircut to elongate the facial shape.

Identify your best facial features and choose a haircut that accentuates those features.

And remember the best haircut for you is the one that makes you feel confident and beautiful!

HAIR TEXTURE

Hair texture describes the circumference of your hair shaft. There are three different hair textures:

- Fine hair texture has a thin hair shaft and is the most fragile. For maximum volume no layers or light layers work best. Careful not to weigh down hair with too much hair product. Use caution with hot tools and hair chemicals to avoid damage.

- Medium hair texture has a thicker hair shaft and is stronger and more resistant to damage. This is the most common texture and looks great with or without layers. Medium hair texture handles hot tools and hair chemicals well.

- Thick hair texture has the thickest hair shaft and is the most resistant to damage. You might want to choose a layered haircut to prevent excessive volume. Hot tools and hair chemicals have to work a little harder to handle this thick hair texture.

HAIR TYPES

Hair type describes whether you have straight hair, wavy hair, curly hair or coily hair.

We can temporarily change our hair type from straight hair to curly hair or from curly hair to straight hair with hot tools like curling irons, flat irons, hot rollers, etc.

For a longer lasting change we have options like permanent waves and hair straightening treatments.

Each hair type has their own maintenance requirements. Choose products made for your specific hair type and desired style.

- Foams and mousses are great for volume and curls and will not weight down your hair.

- Gels come in light hold to strong hold and are great for controlling your hair into a desired style.

- Leave-in conditioners will moisturize and protect your hair from damage.

- Heat protectants will add a barrier between your hair and hot tools.

- Hair spray comes in light hold to strong hold and helps your hairstyle stay in place.

Chapter 1
THE OVAL HAIRCUT

This super sexy haircut has a lot to offer. It is very flattering and versatile.

- **LENGTH-** The Oval Haircut looks great in short lengths, medium lengths, and long lengths.

- **PART-** This haircut has a changeable part.

- **BANGS-** The bangs can be shorter or longer to suit your personal preference.

- **LAYERS-** Choose short layers, long layers or no layers to serve your unique hair texture and hair type.

- **STYLING-** The Oval Haircut has many styling options. Style your hair straight or curled, up or down, and everyway in between. Longer lengths look great in updo's, ponytails and braids.

THE OVAL HAIRCUT

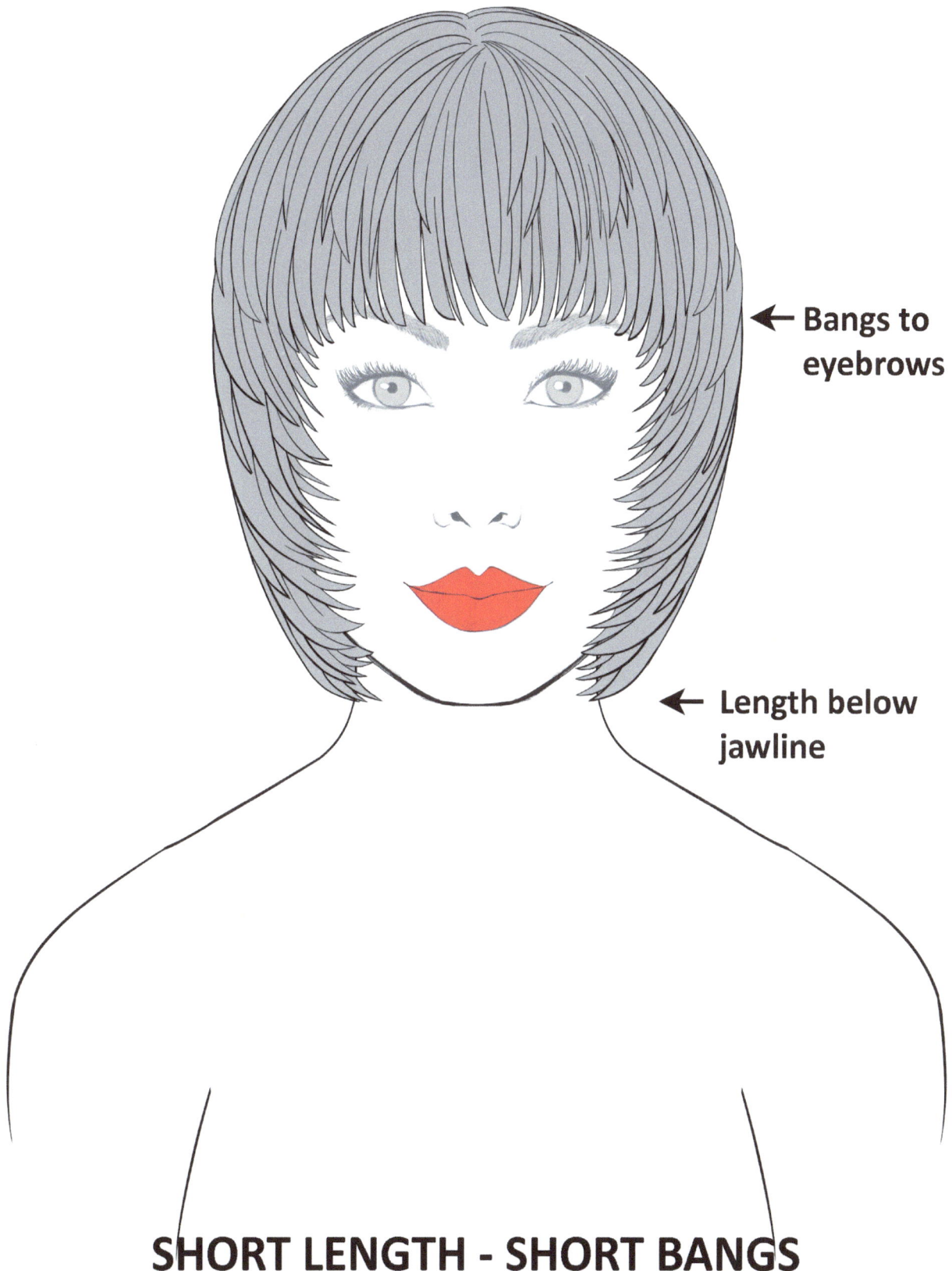

← **Bangs to eyebrows**

← **Length below jawline**

SHORT LENGTH - SHORT BANGS

THE OVAL HAIRCUT

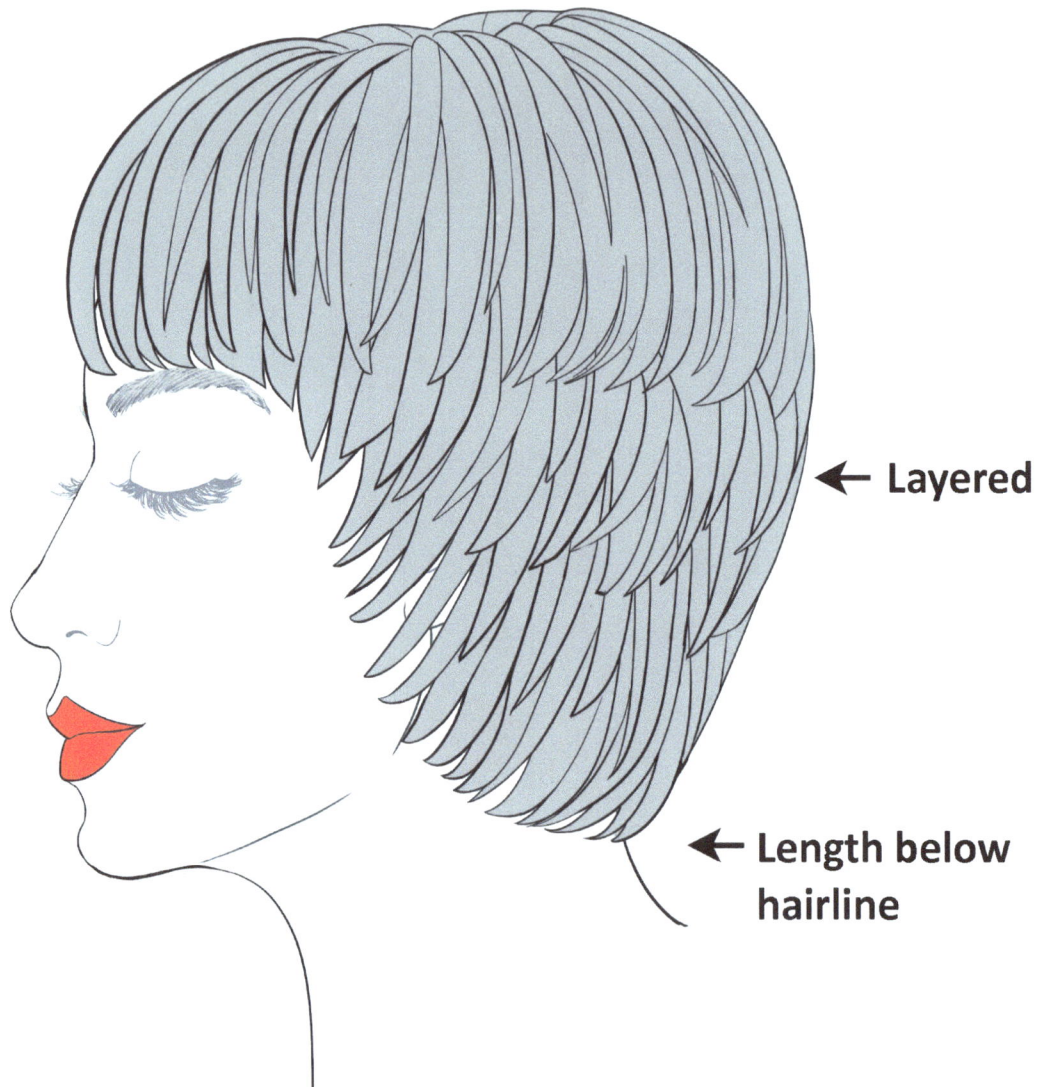

← Layered

← Length below
hairline

SHORT LENGTH - SHORT BANGS

THE OVAL HAIRCUT

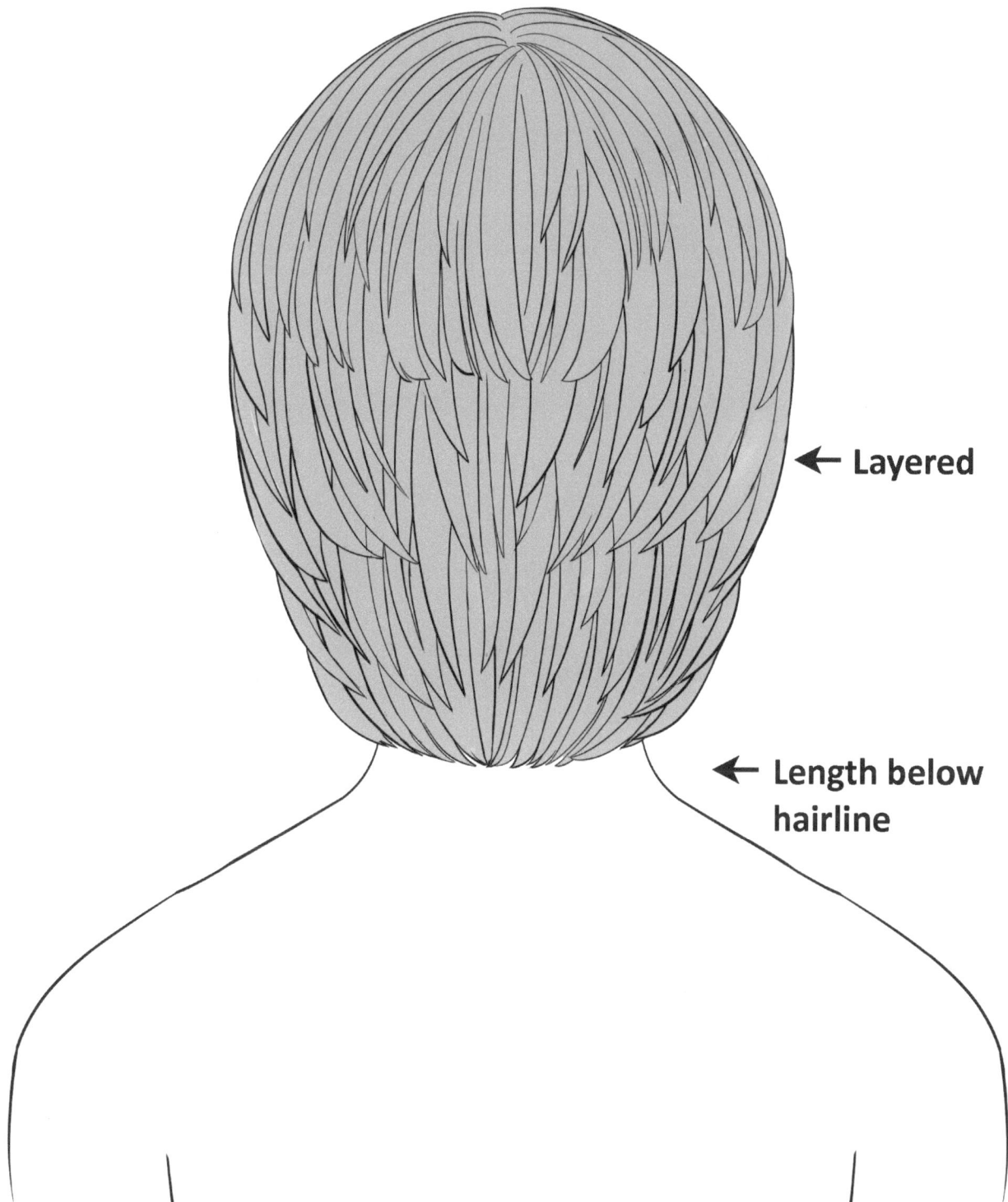

← Layered

← Length below
hairline

SHORT LENGTH - SHORT BANGS

THE OVAL HAIRCUT

Styling Options

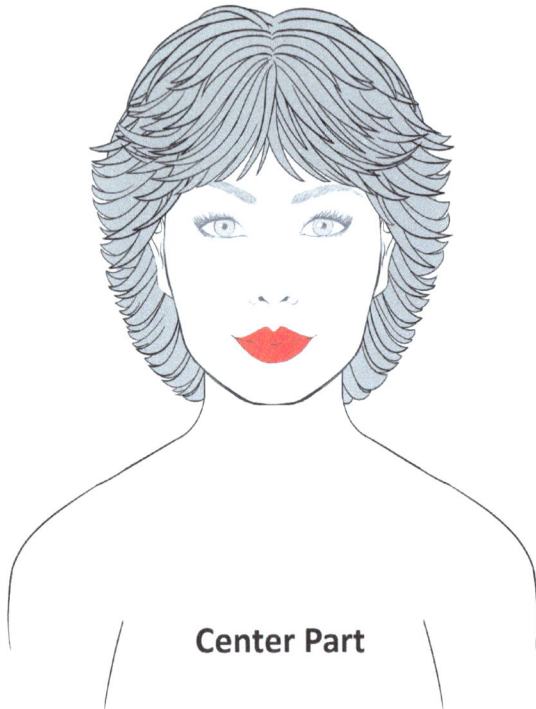

Center Part

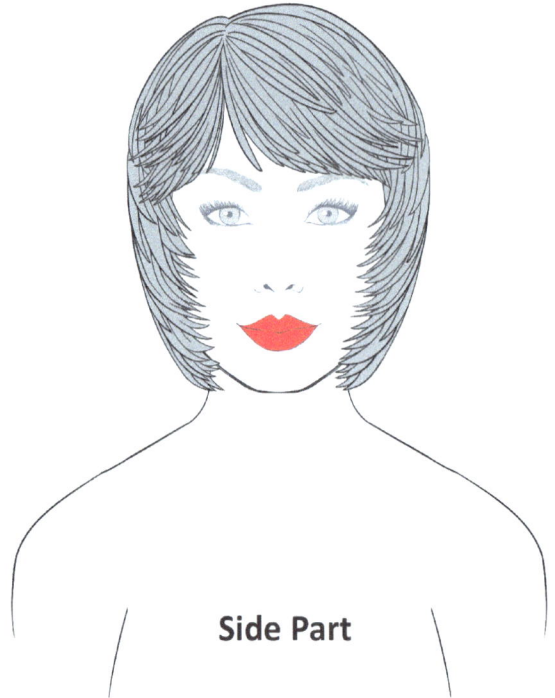

Side Part

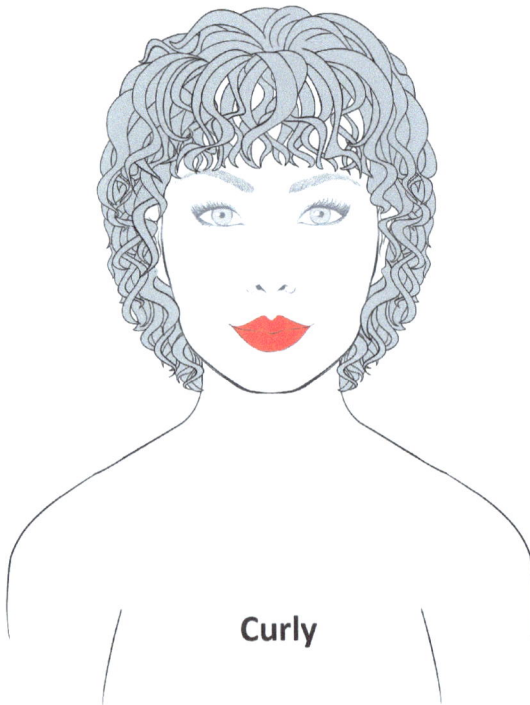

Curly

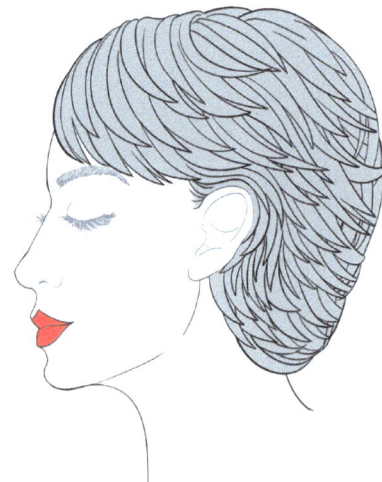

Away From Ears

SHORT LENGTH - SHORT BANGS

THE OVAL HAIRCUT

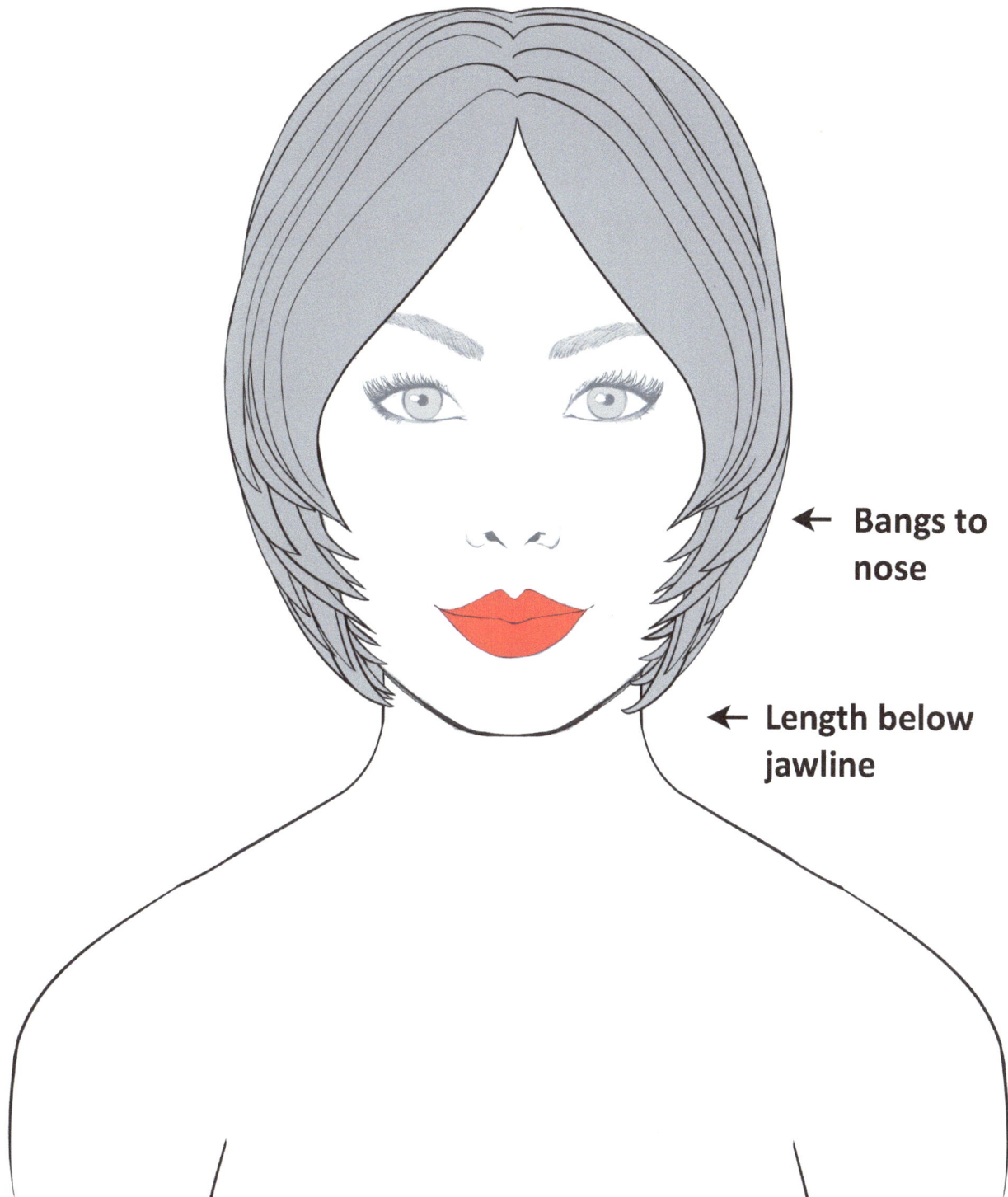

← **Bangs to nose**

← **Length below jawline**

SHORT LENGTH - LONG BANGS

THE OVAL HAIRCUT

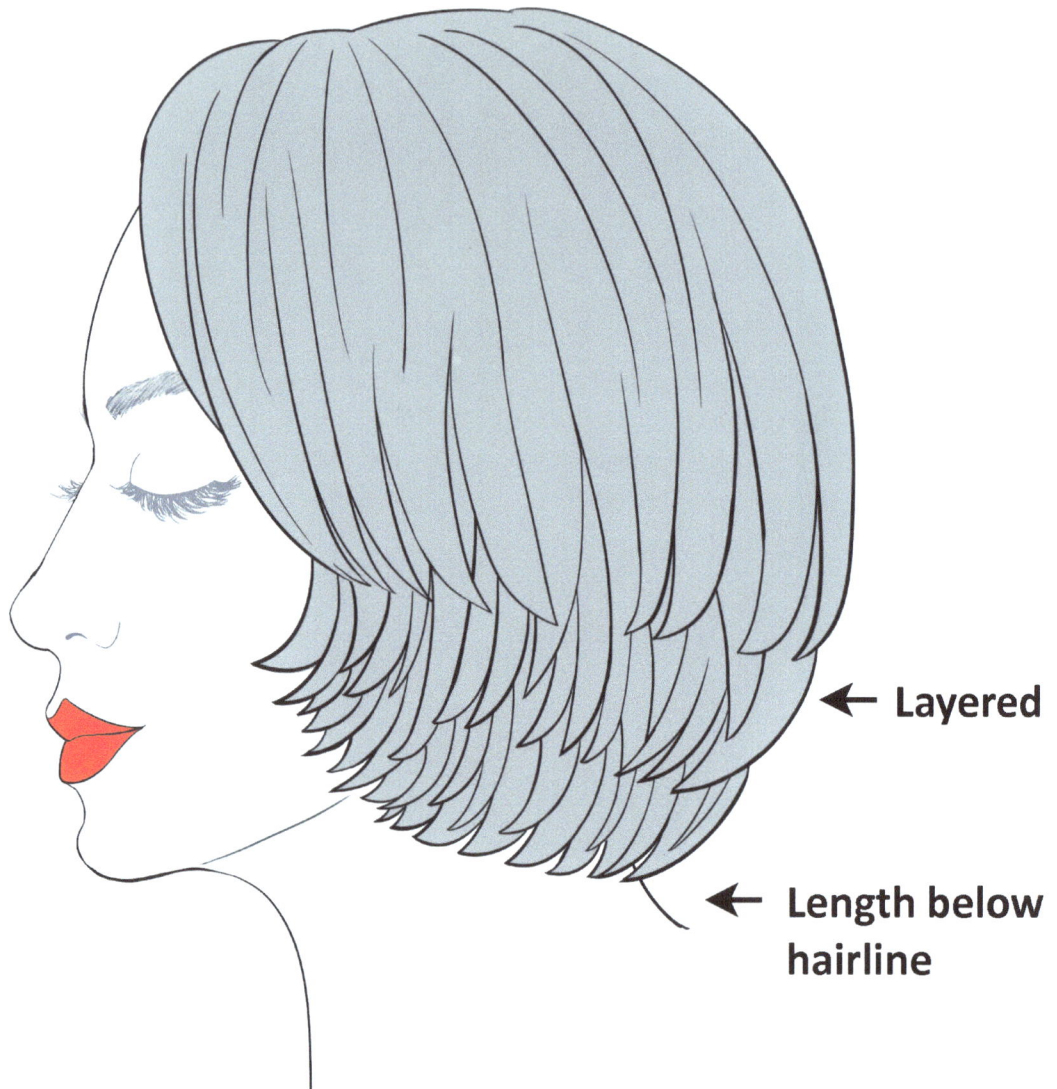

← Layered

← Length below
hairline

SHORT LENGTH - LONG BANGS

THE OVAL HAIRCUT

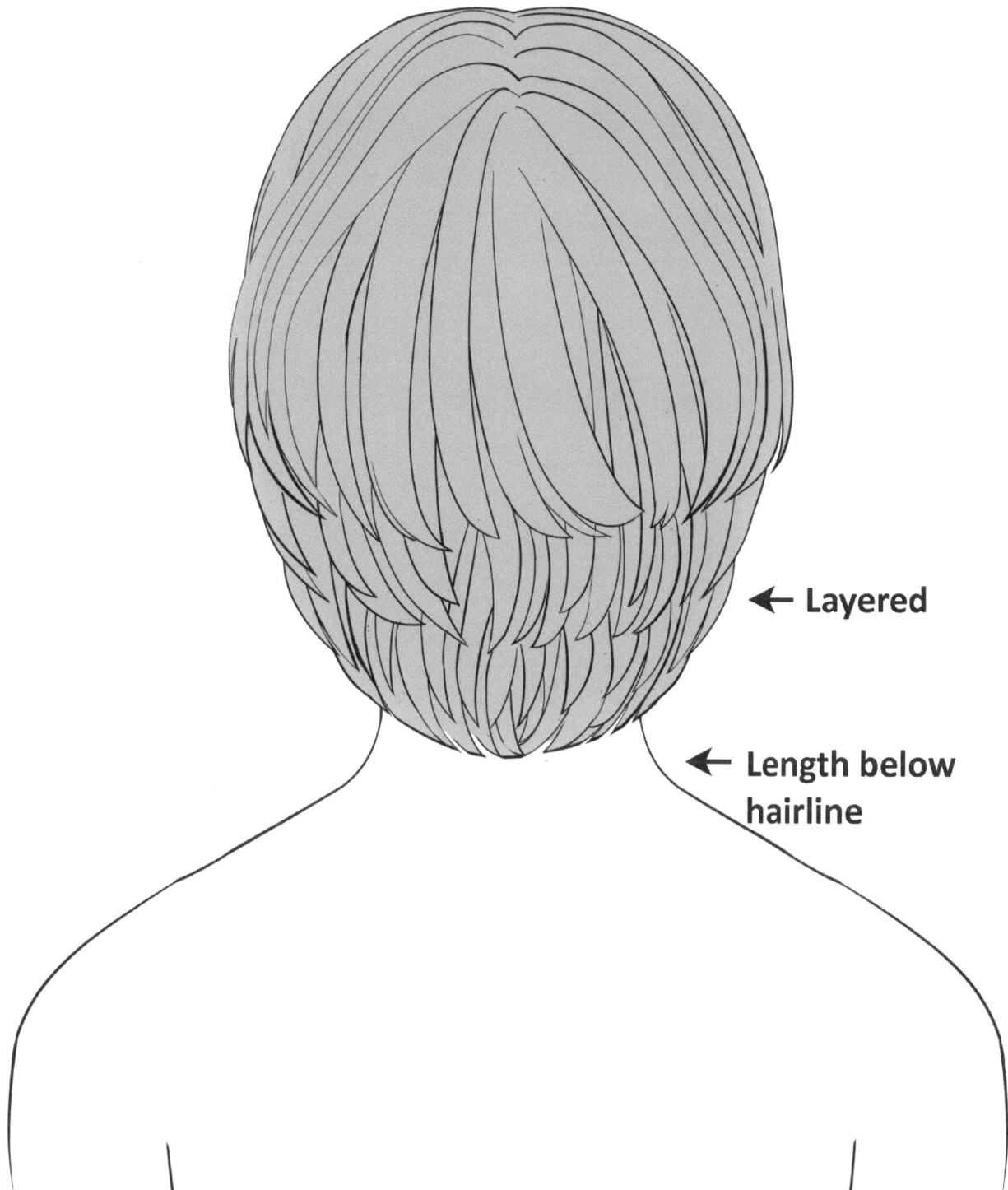

← Layered

← Length below
hairline

SHORT LENGTH - LONG BANGS

THE OVAL HAIRCUT

Styling Options

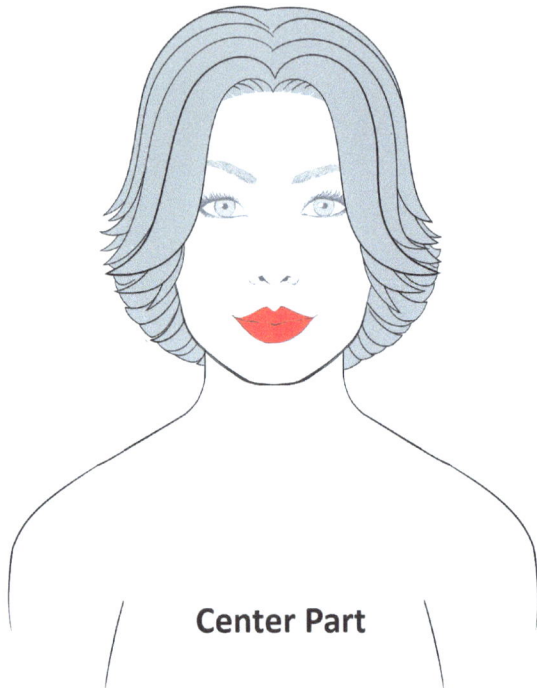

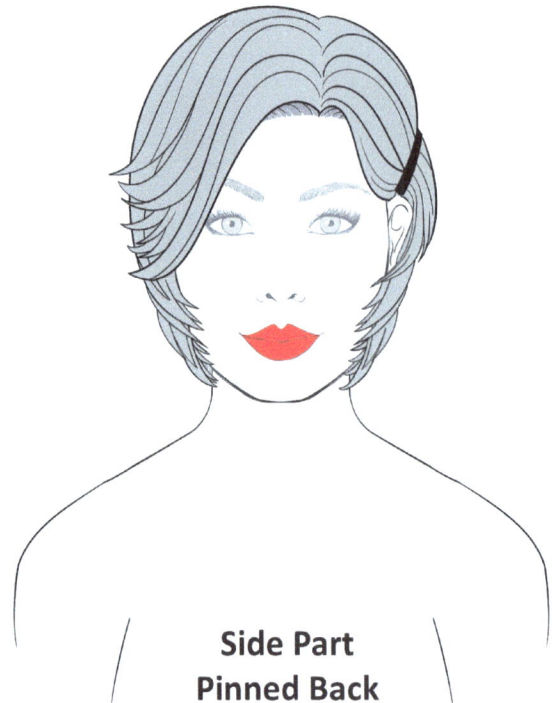

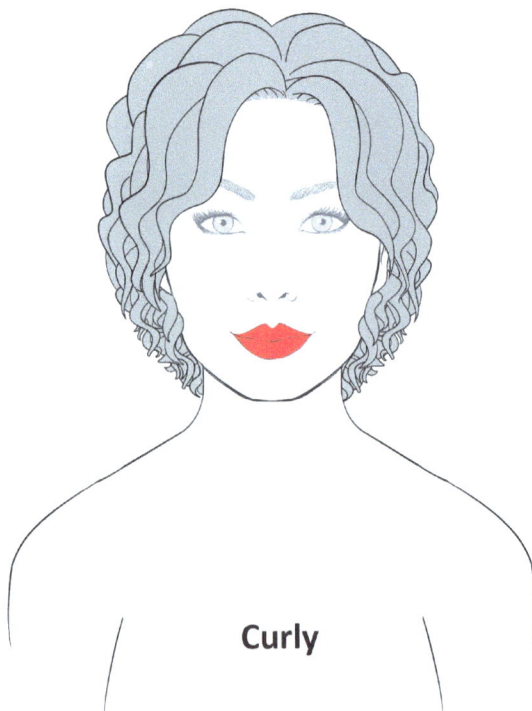

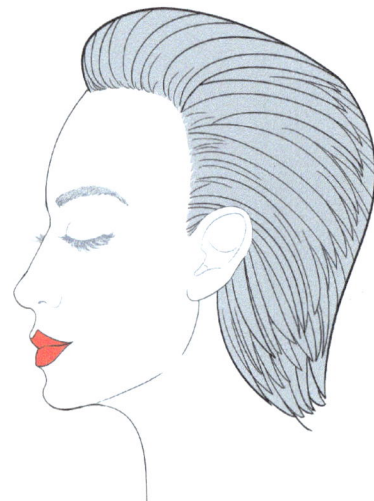

Center Part

**Side Part
Pinned Back**

Curly

Slicked Back

SHORT LENGTH - LONG BANGS

THE OVAL HAIRCUT

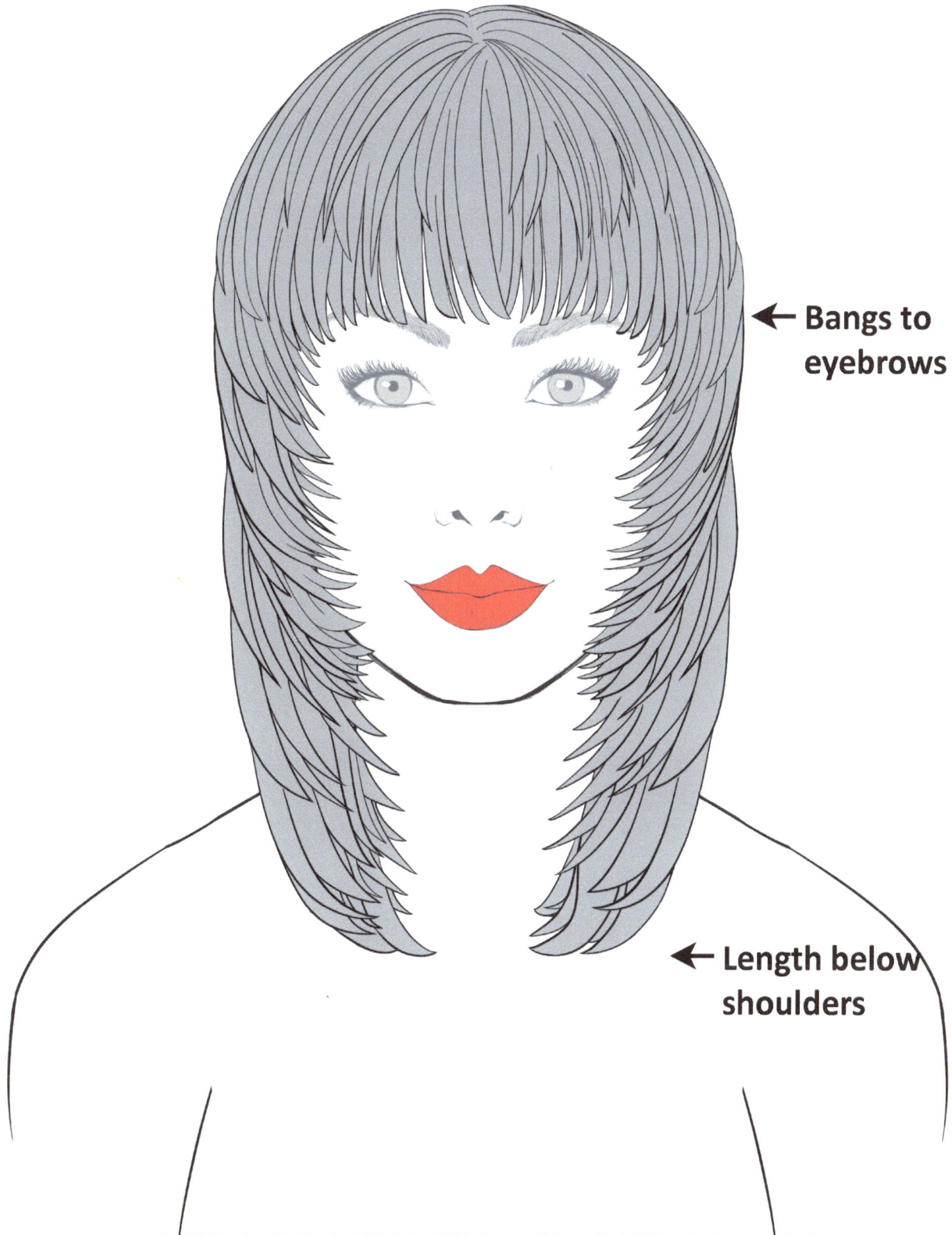

← **Bangs to eyebrows**

← **Length below shoulders**

MEDIUM LENGTH - SHORT BANGS

THE OVAL HAIRCUT

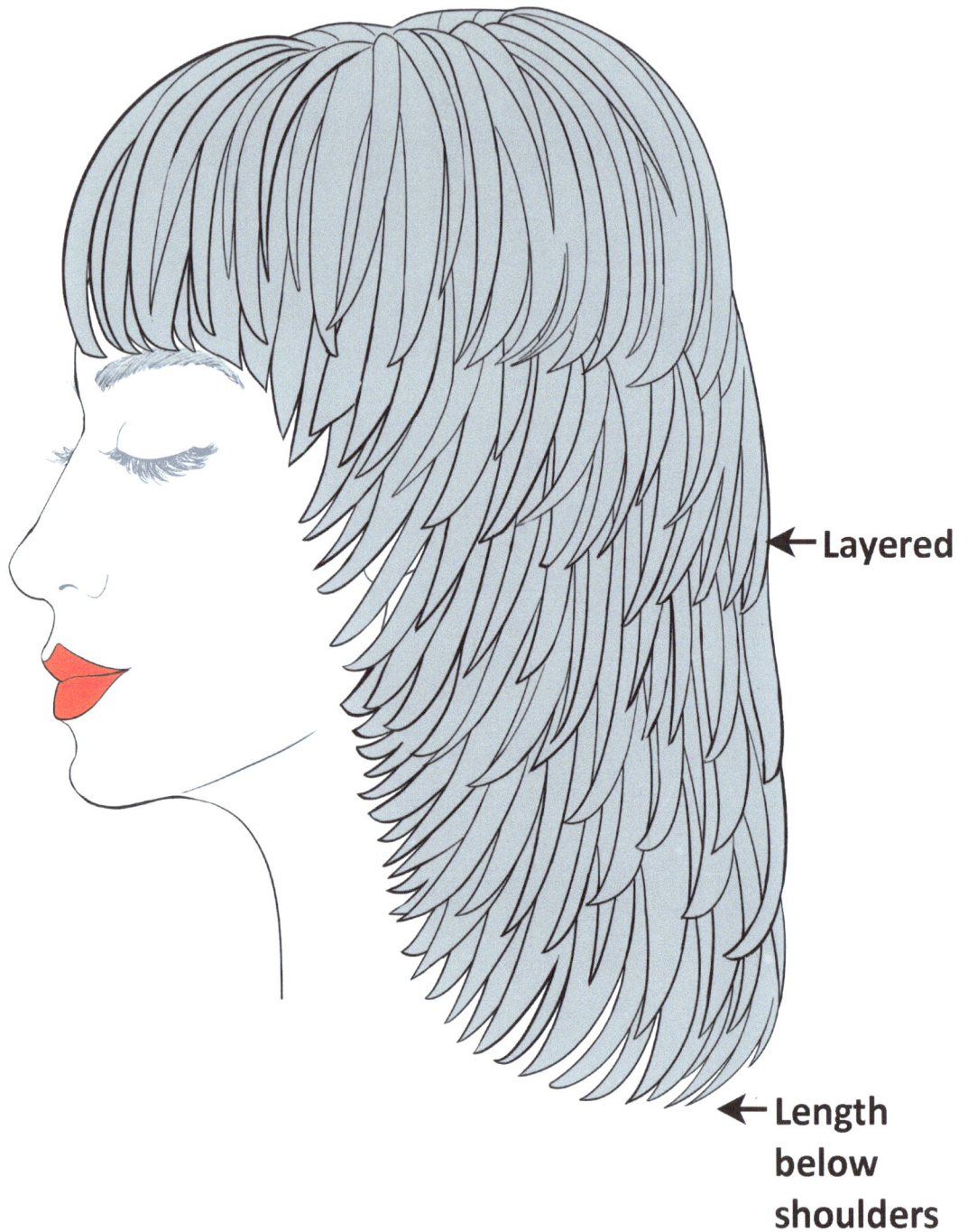

← Layered

← Length
below
shoulders

MEDIUM LENGTH - SHORT BANGS

THE OVAL HAIRCUT

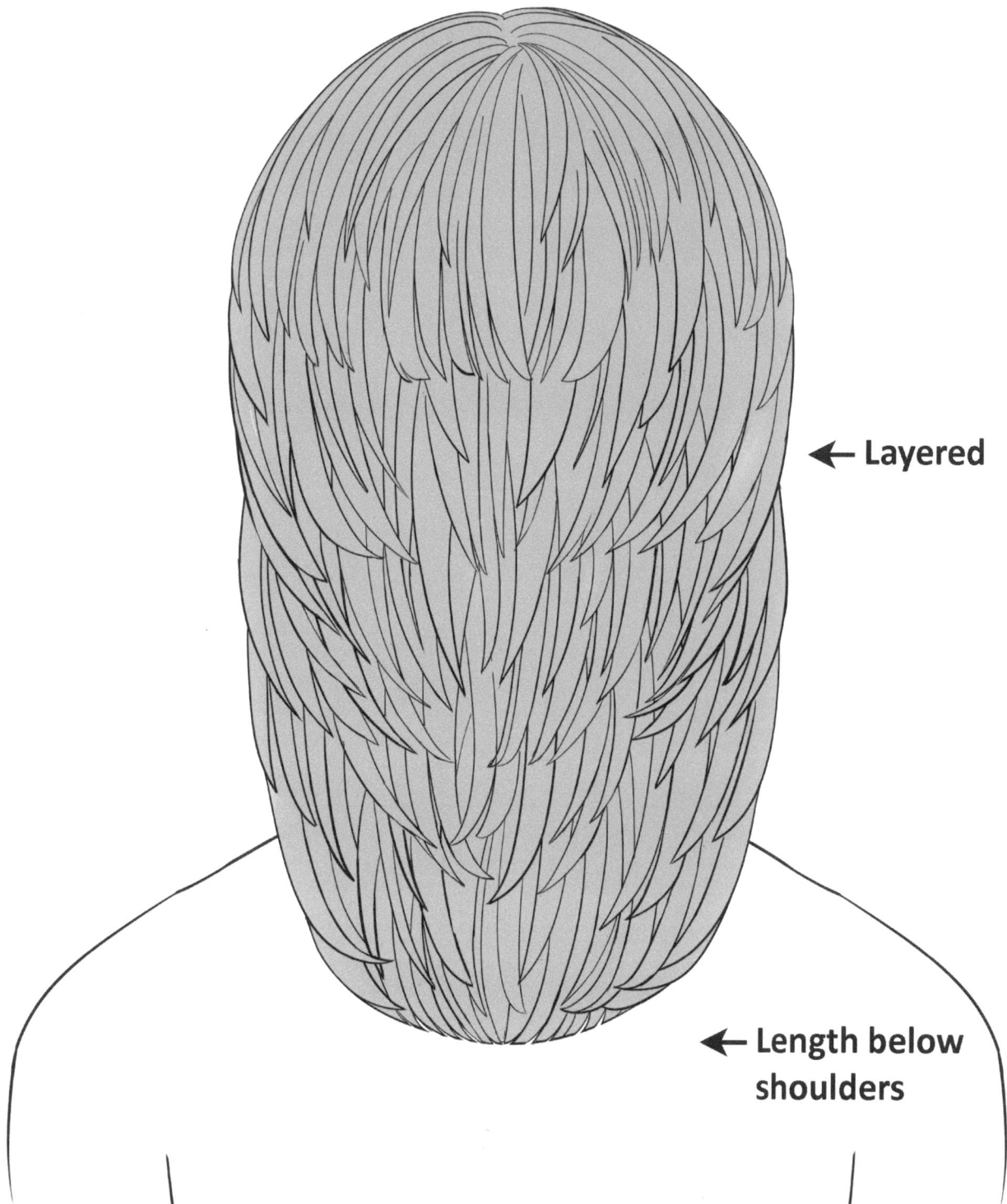

← Layered

← Length below shoulders

MEDIUM LENGTH - SHORT BANGS

THE OVAL HAIRCUT

Styling Options

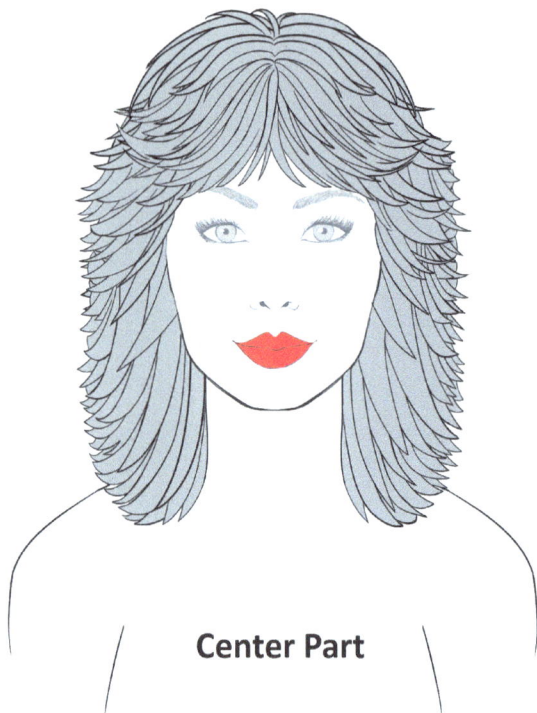

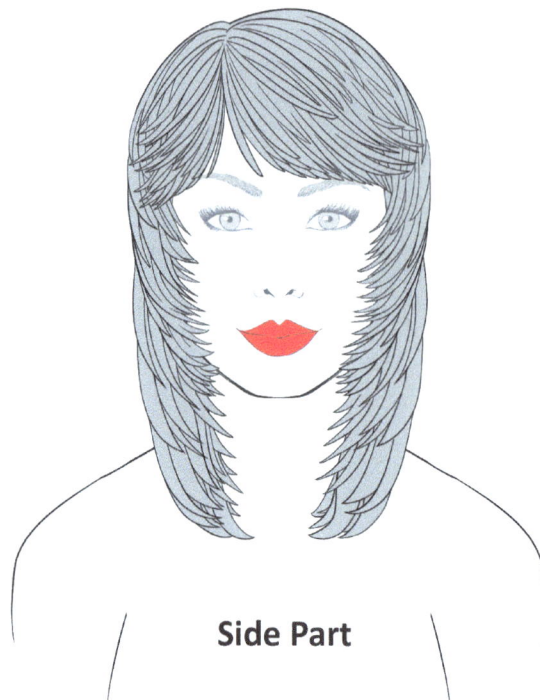

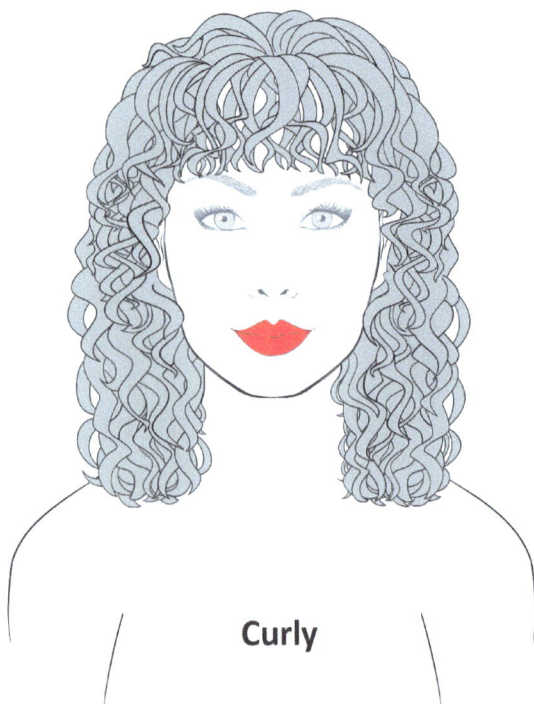

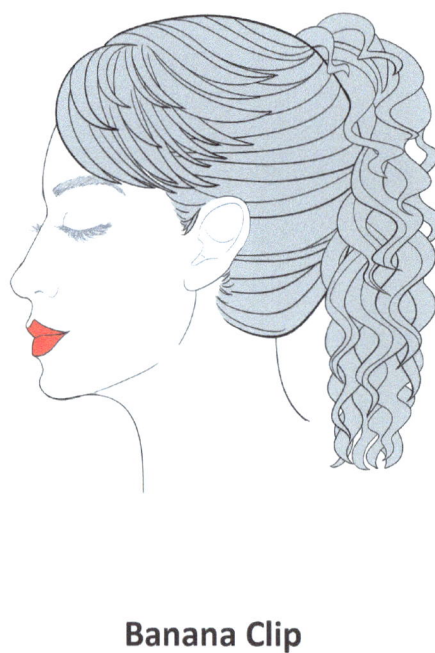

Center Part

Side Part

Curly

Banana Clip

MEDIUM LENGTH - SHORT BANGS

THE OVAL HAIRCUT

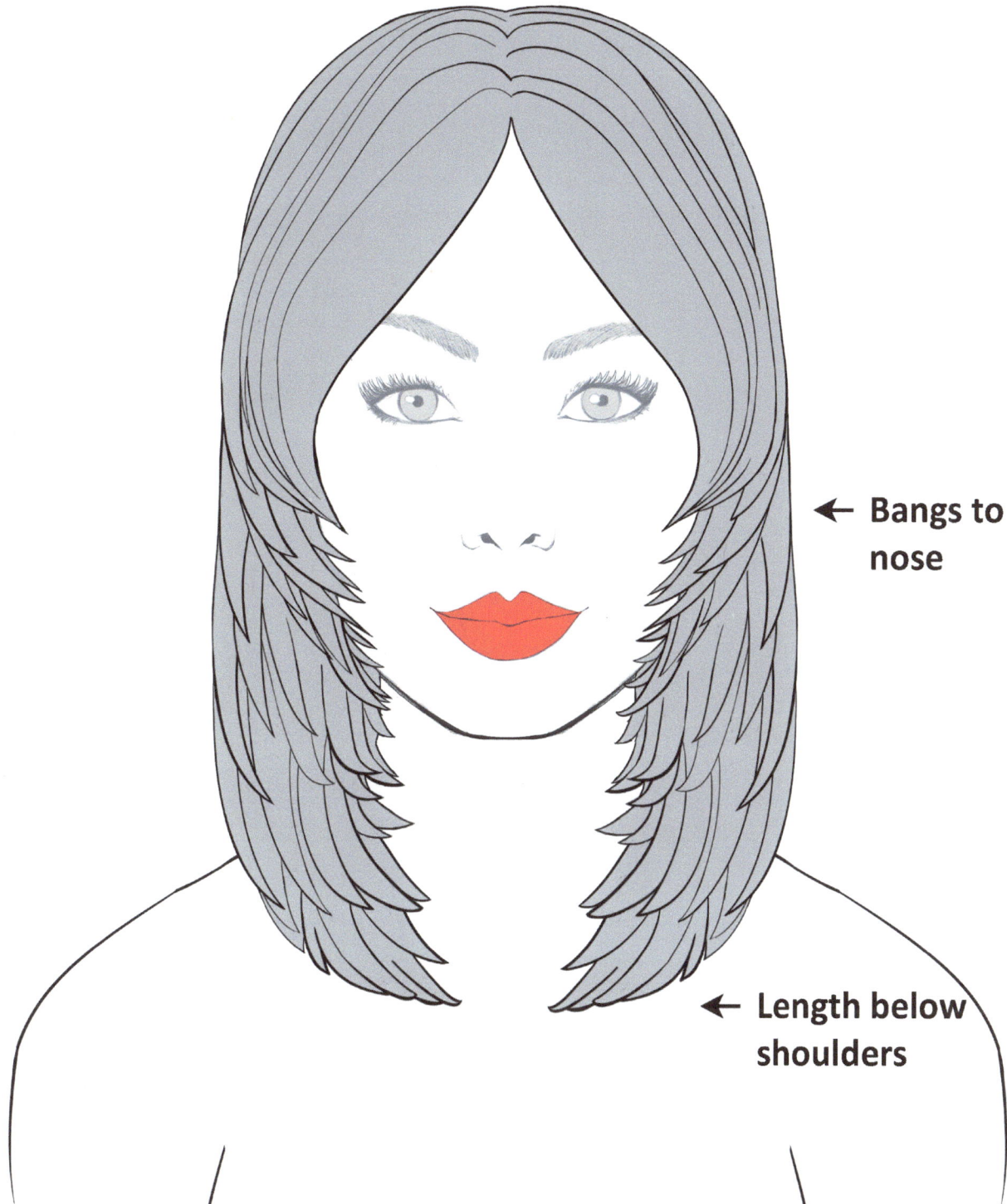

← **Bangs to nose**

← **Length below shoulders**

MEDIUM LENGTH - LONG BANGS

THE OVAL HAIRCUT

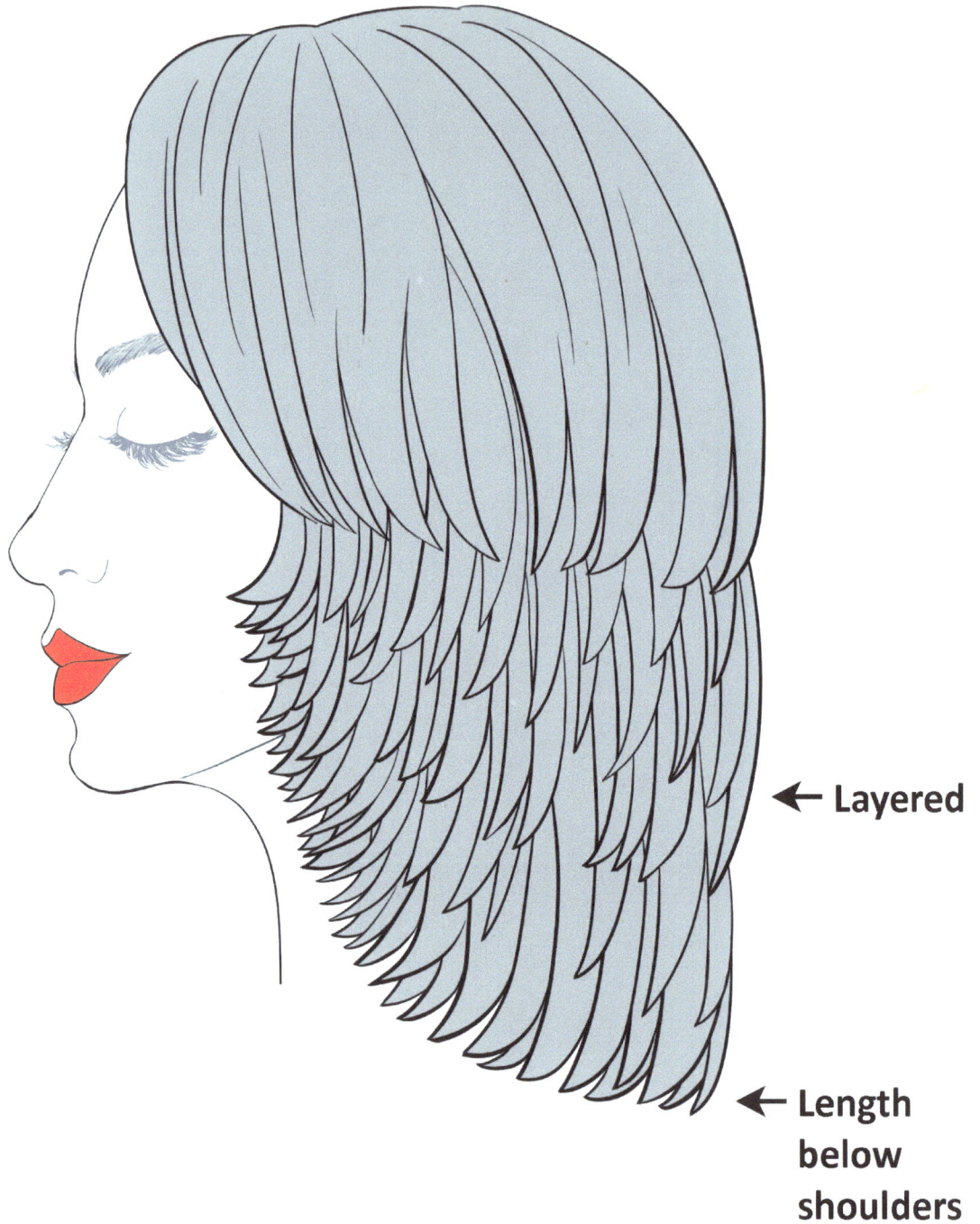

← Layered

← Length below shoulders

MEDIUM LENGTH - LONG BANGS

THE OVAL HAIRCUT

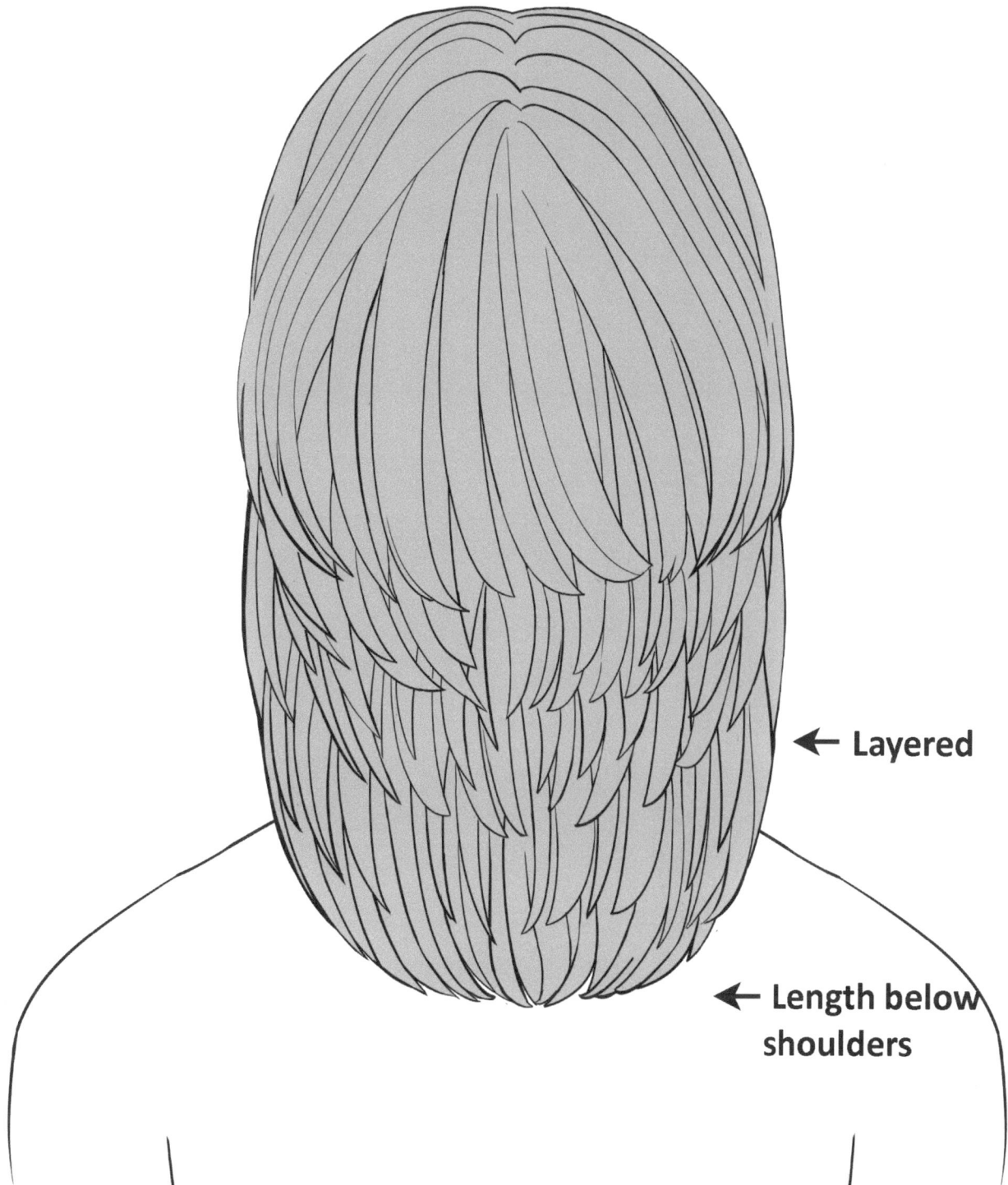

← Layered

← Length below shoulders

MEDIUM LENGTH - LONG BANGS

THE OVAL HAIRCUT

Styling Options

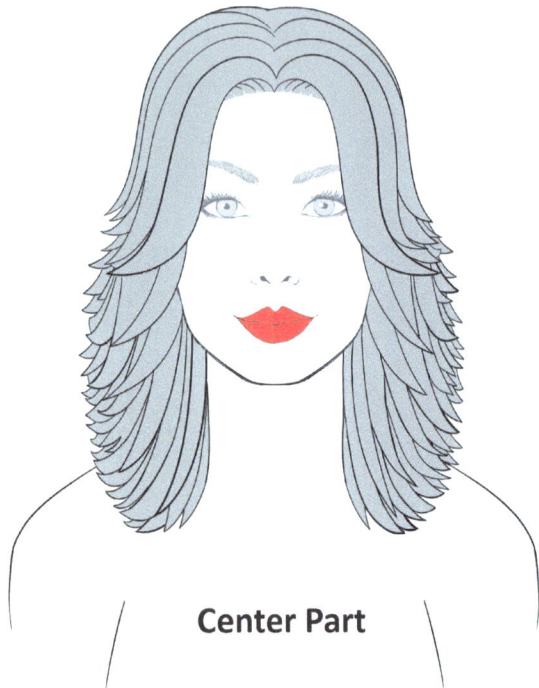

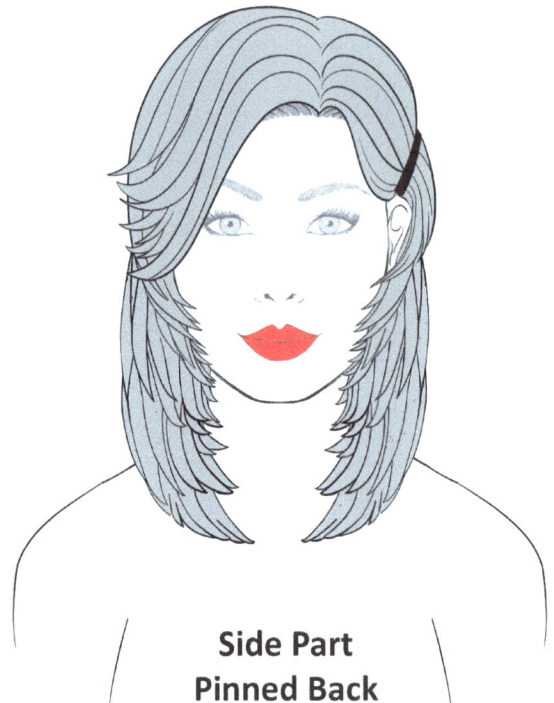

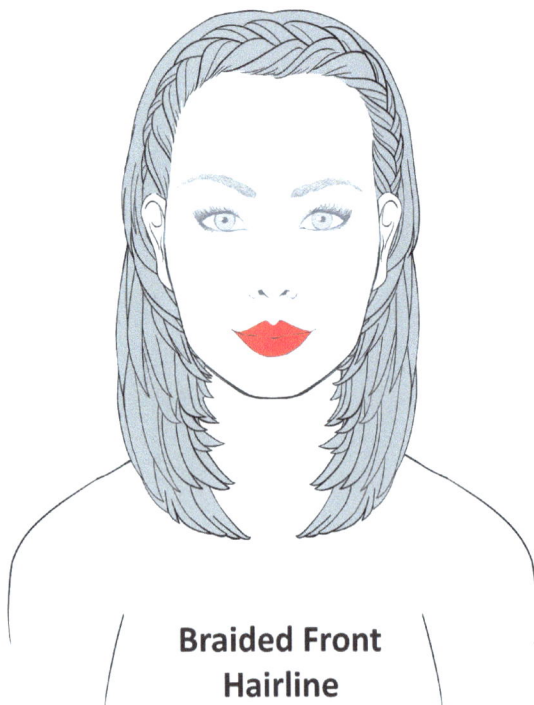

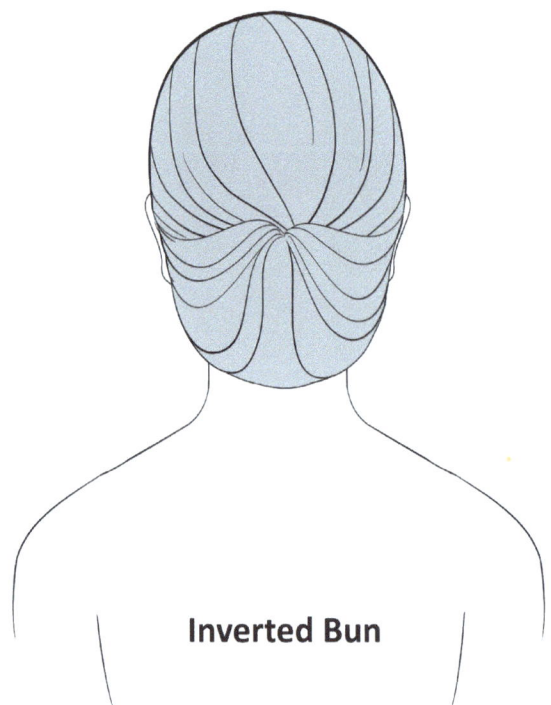

Center Part

**Side Part
Pinned Back**

**Braided Front
Hairline**

Inverted Bun

MEDIUM LENGTH - LONG BANGS

THE OVAL HAIRCUT

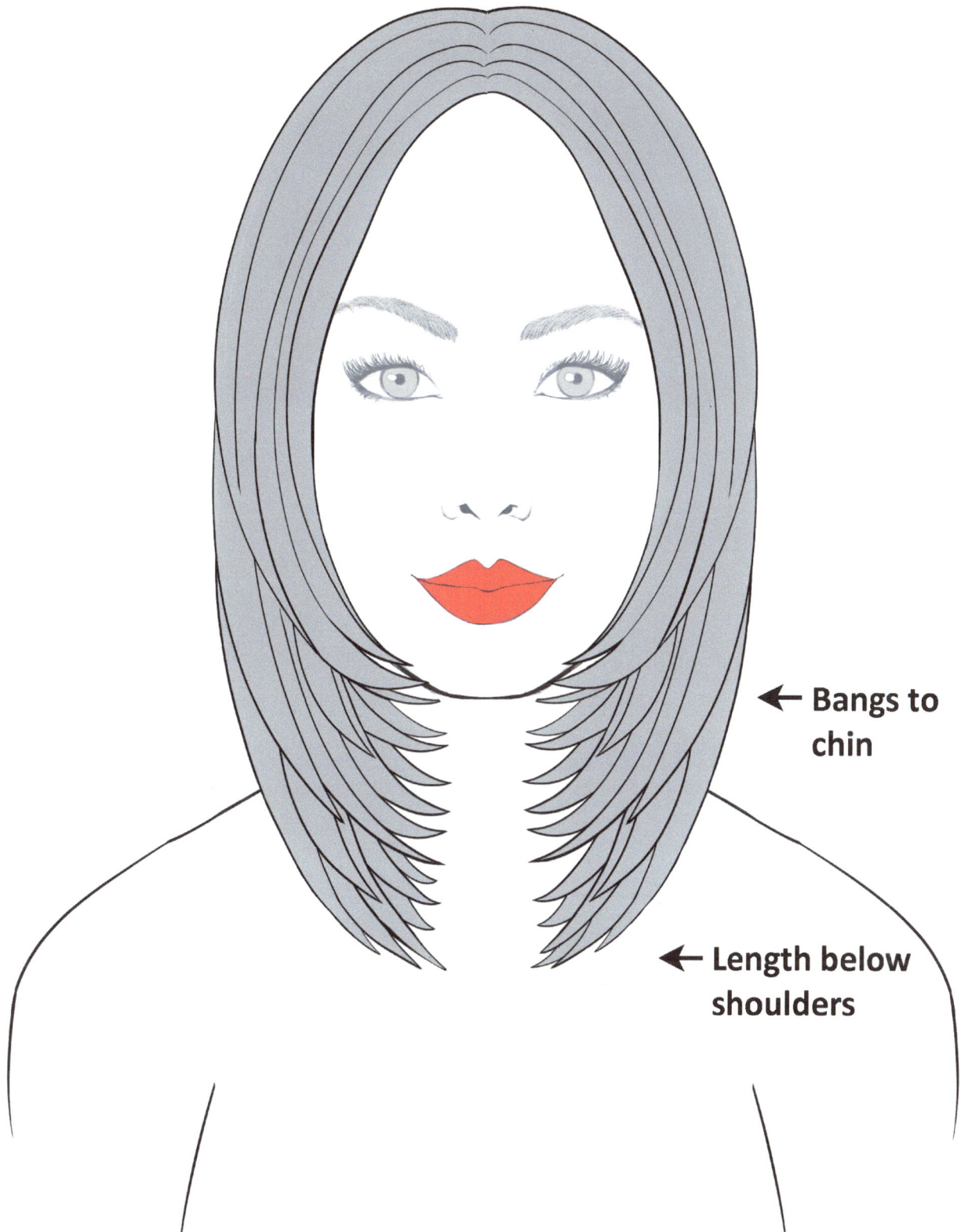

← **Bangs to chin**

← **Length below shoulders**

MEDIUM LENGTH - BANGS TO CHIN

THE OVAL HAIRCUT

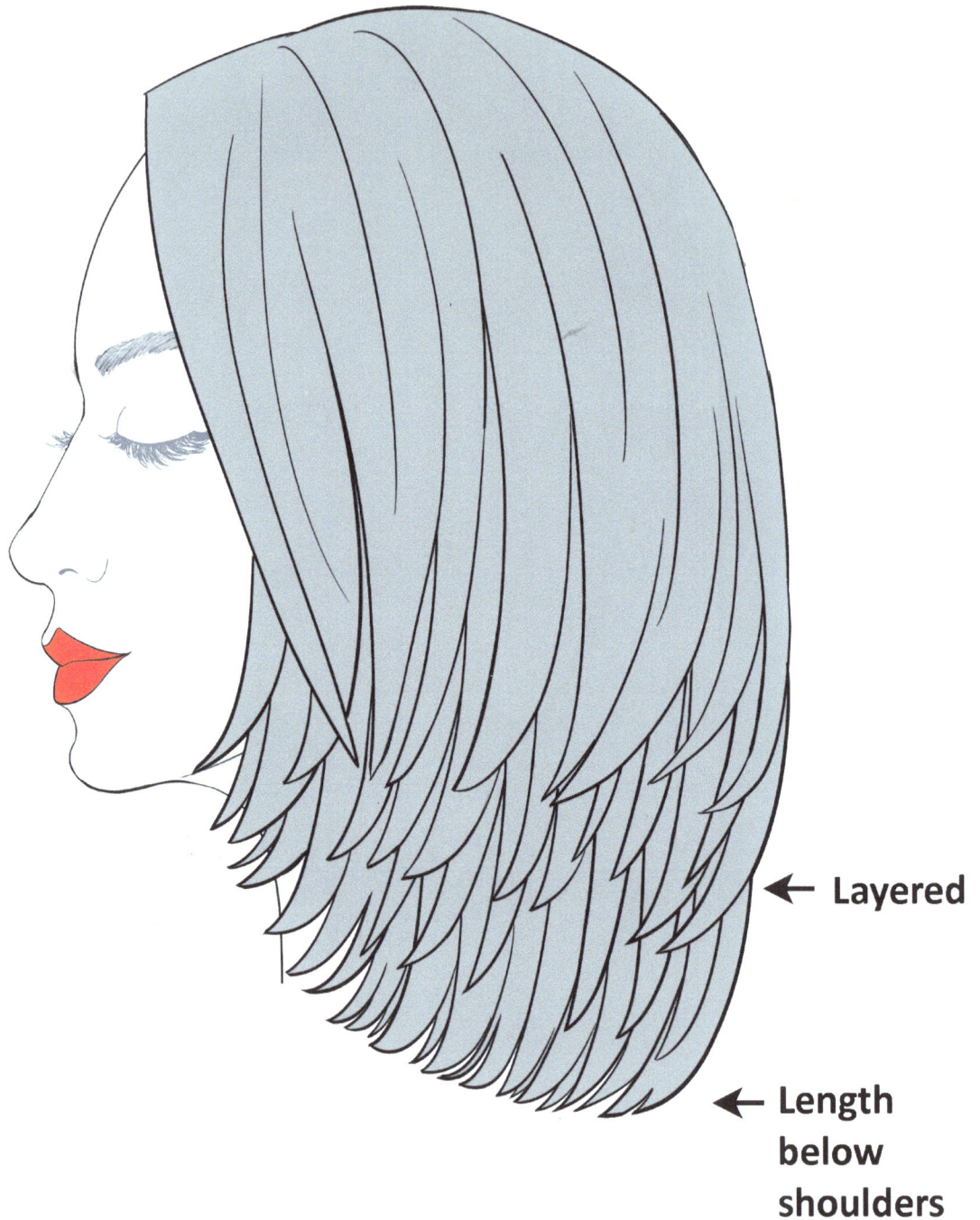

← Layered

← Length below shoulders

MEDIUM LENGTH - BANGS TO CHIN

THE OVAL HAIRCUT

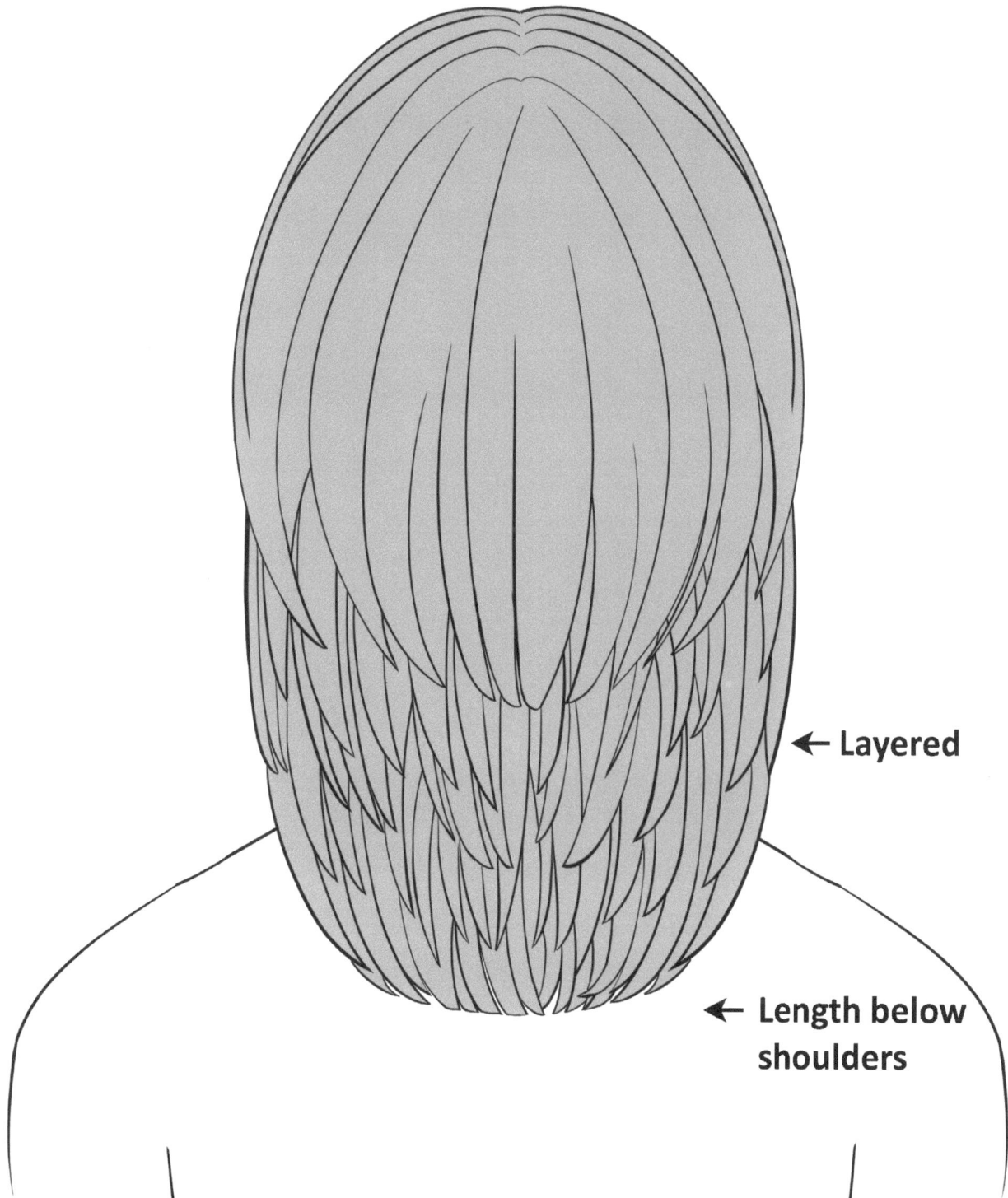

← Layered

← Length below shoulders

MEDIUM LENGTH - BANGS TO CHIN

THE OVAL HAIRCUT

Styling Options

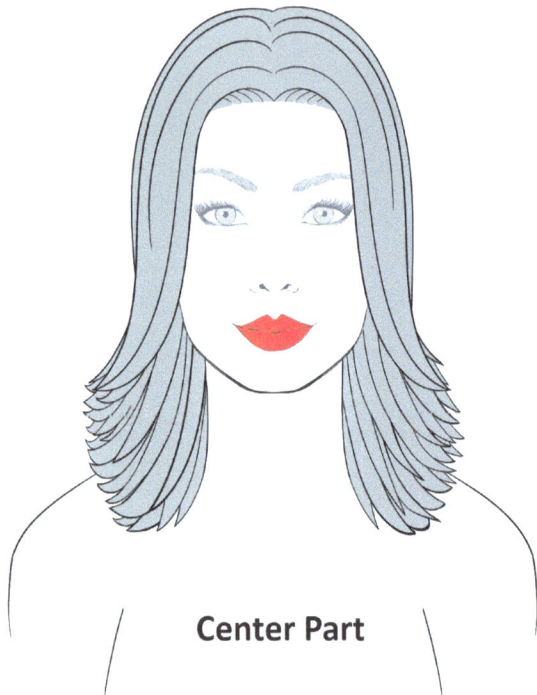

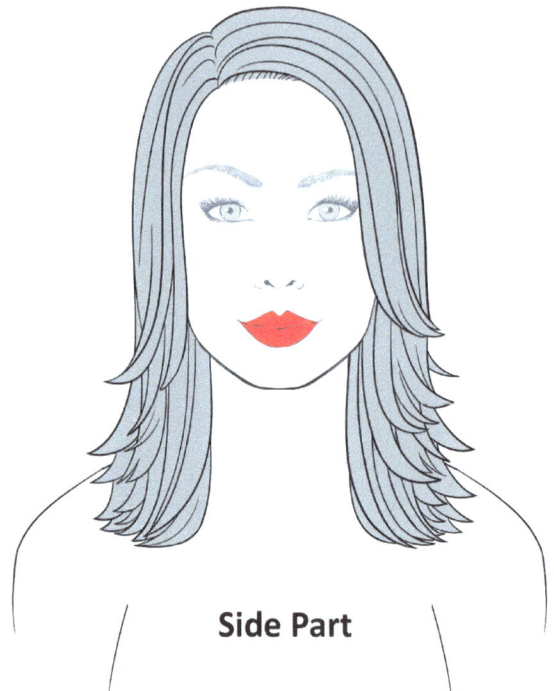

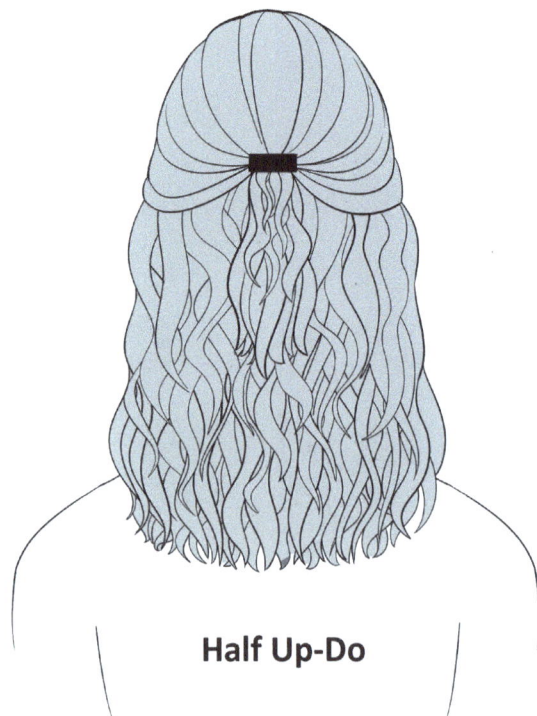

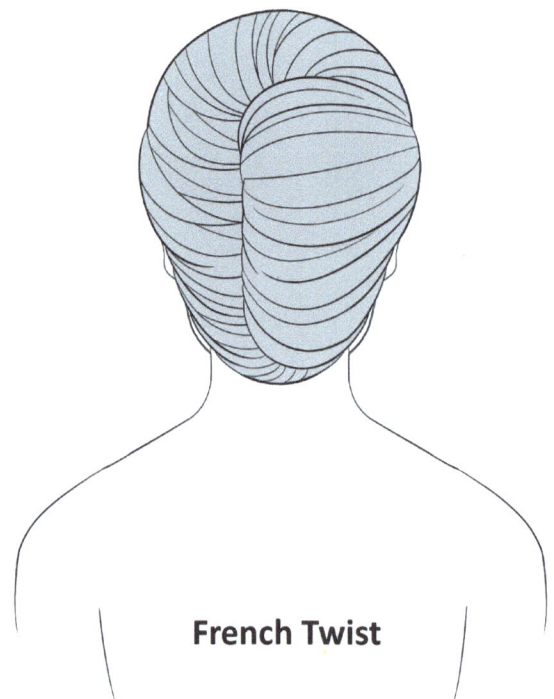

Center Part

Side Part

Half Up-Do

French Twist

MEDIUM LENGTH - BANGS TO CHIN

THE OVAL HAIRCUT

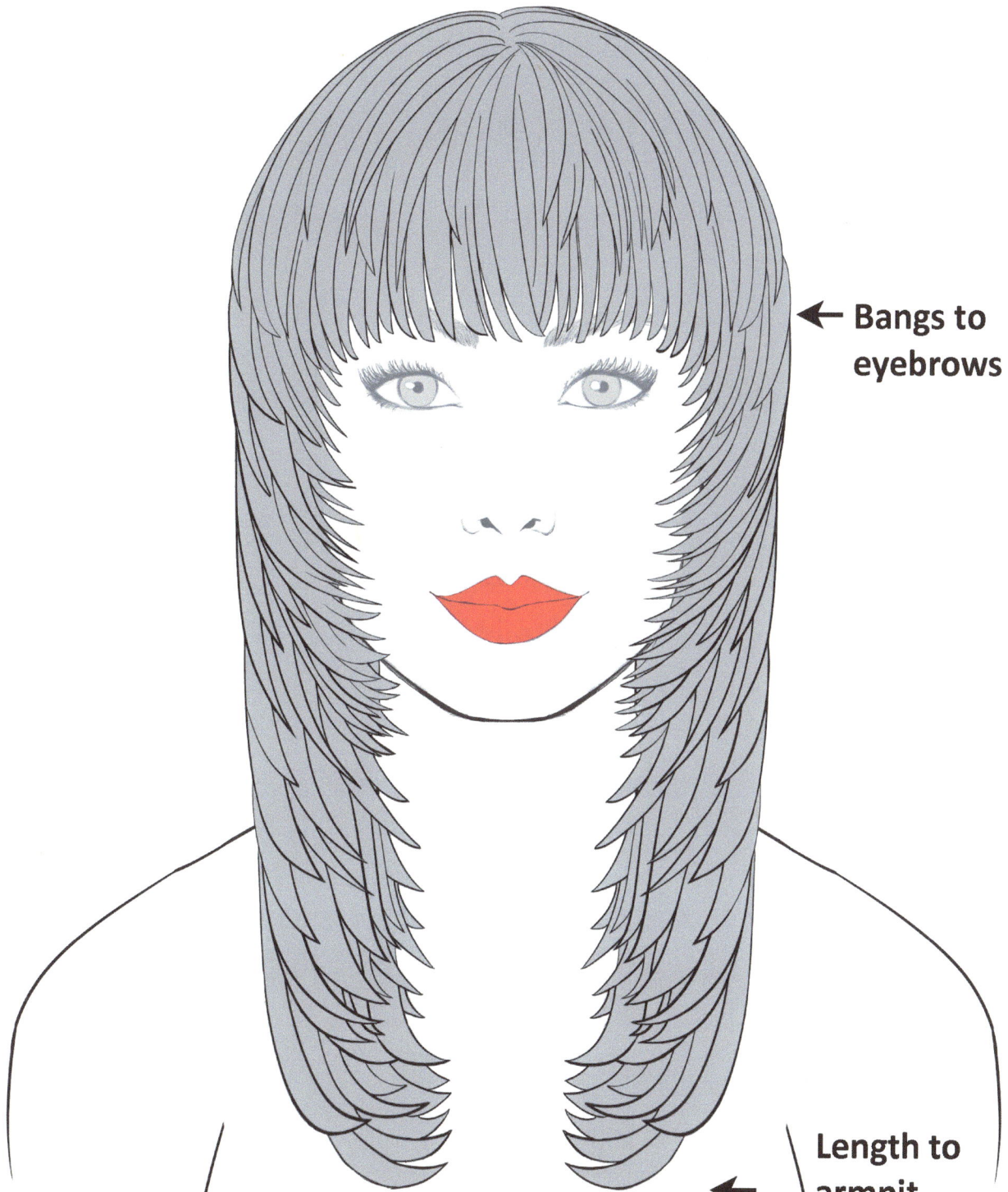

← Bangs to eyebrows

Length to armpit ←

LONG LENGTH - SHORT BANGS

THE OVAL HAIRCUT

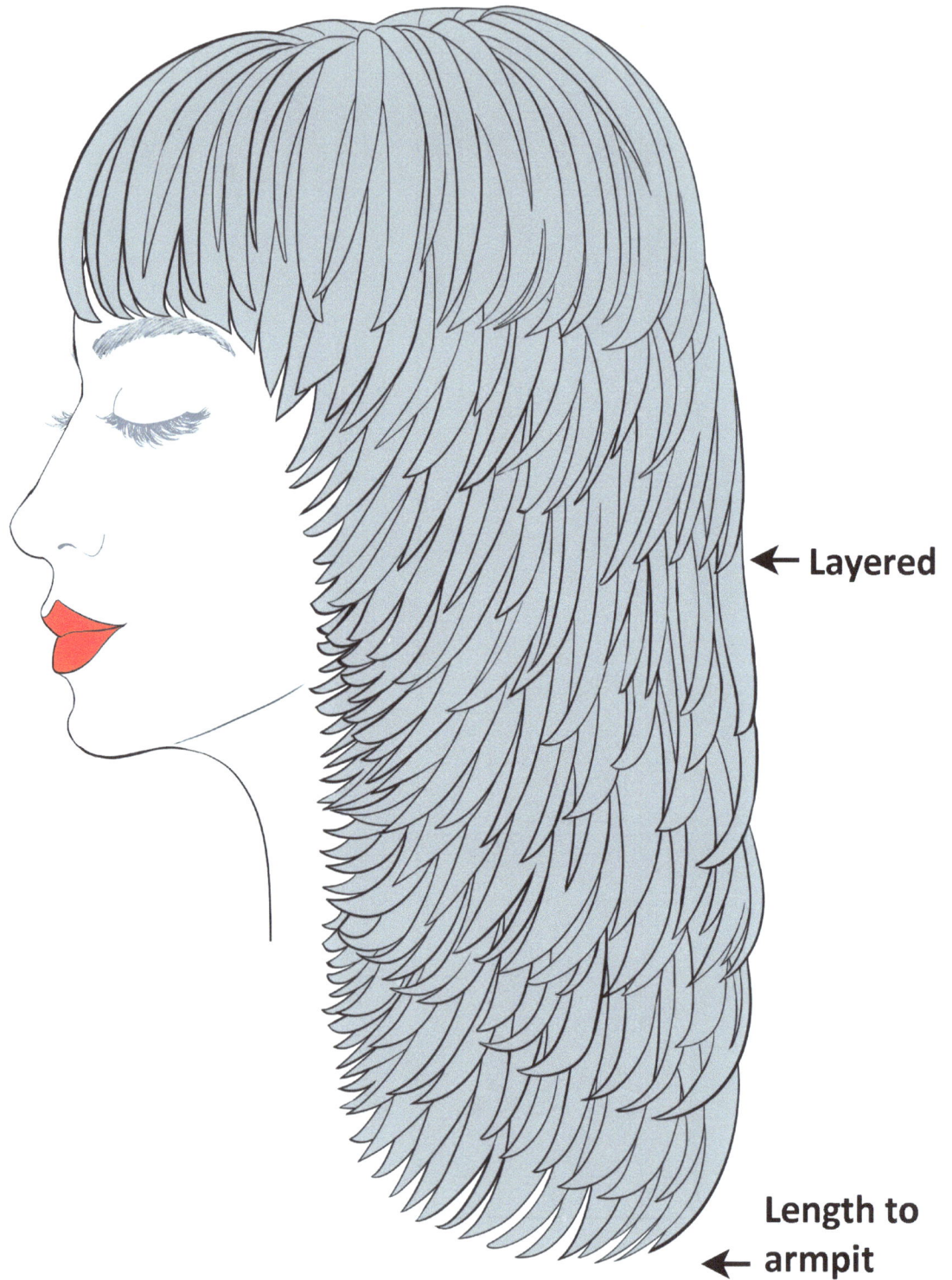

← Layered

Length to
← armpit

LONG LENGTH - SHORT BANGS

THE OVAL HAIRCUT

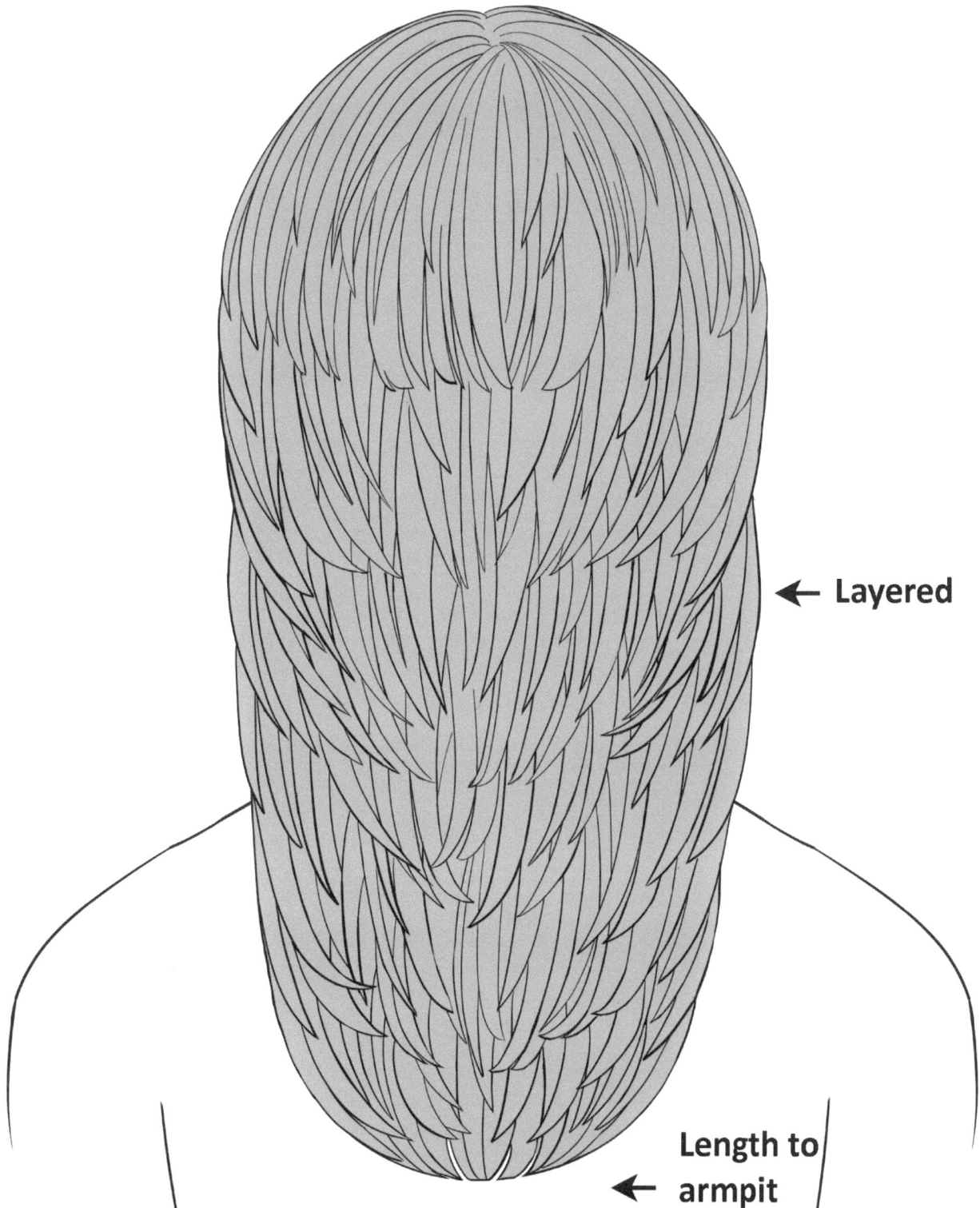

← Layered

Length to
← armpit

LONG LENGTH - SHORT BANGS

THE OVAL HAIRCUT

Styling Options

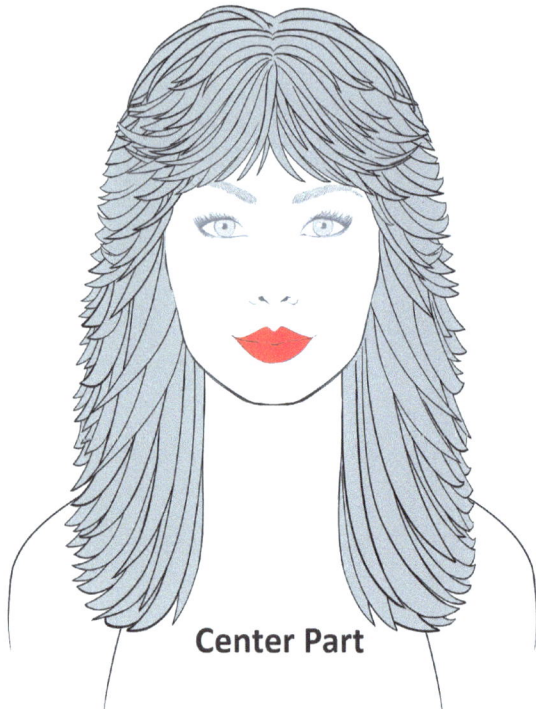

Center Part

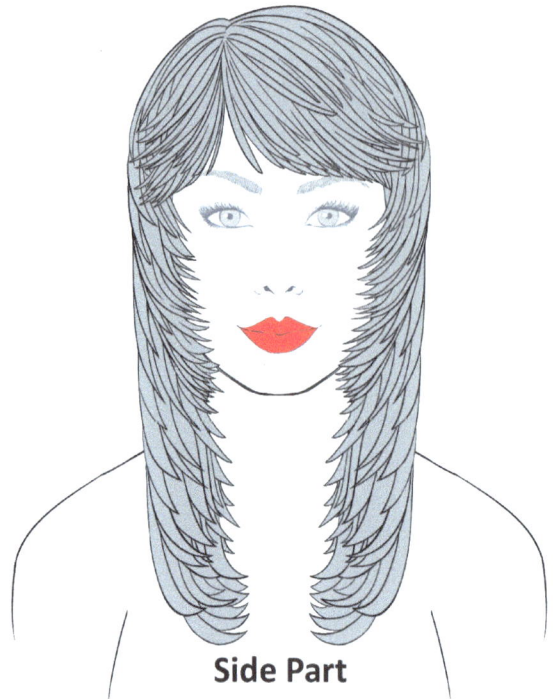

Side Part

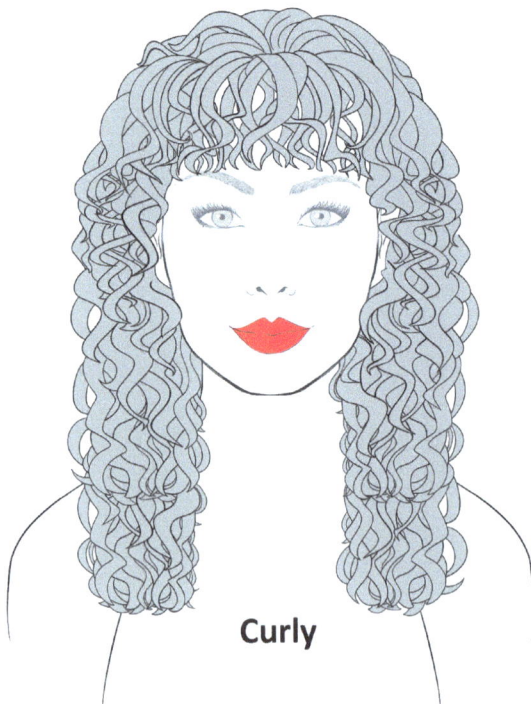

Curly

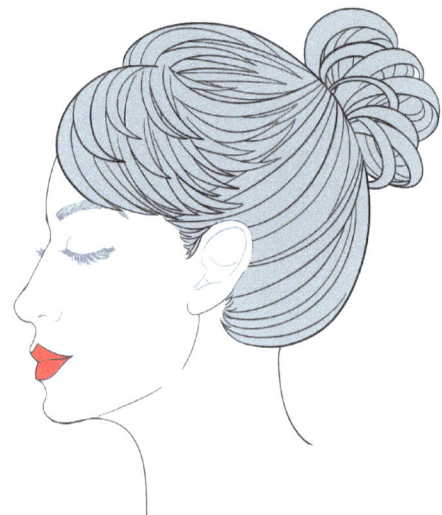

Up-Do

LONG LENGTH - SHORT BANGS

THE OVAL HAIRCUT

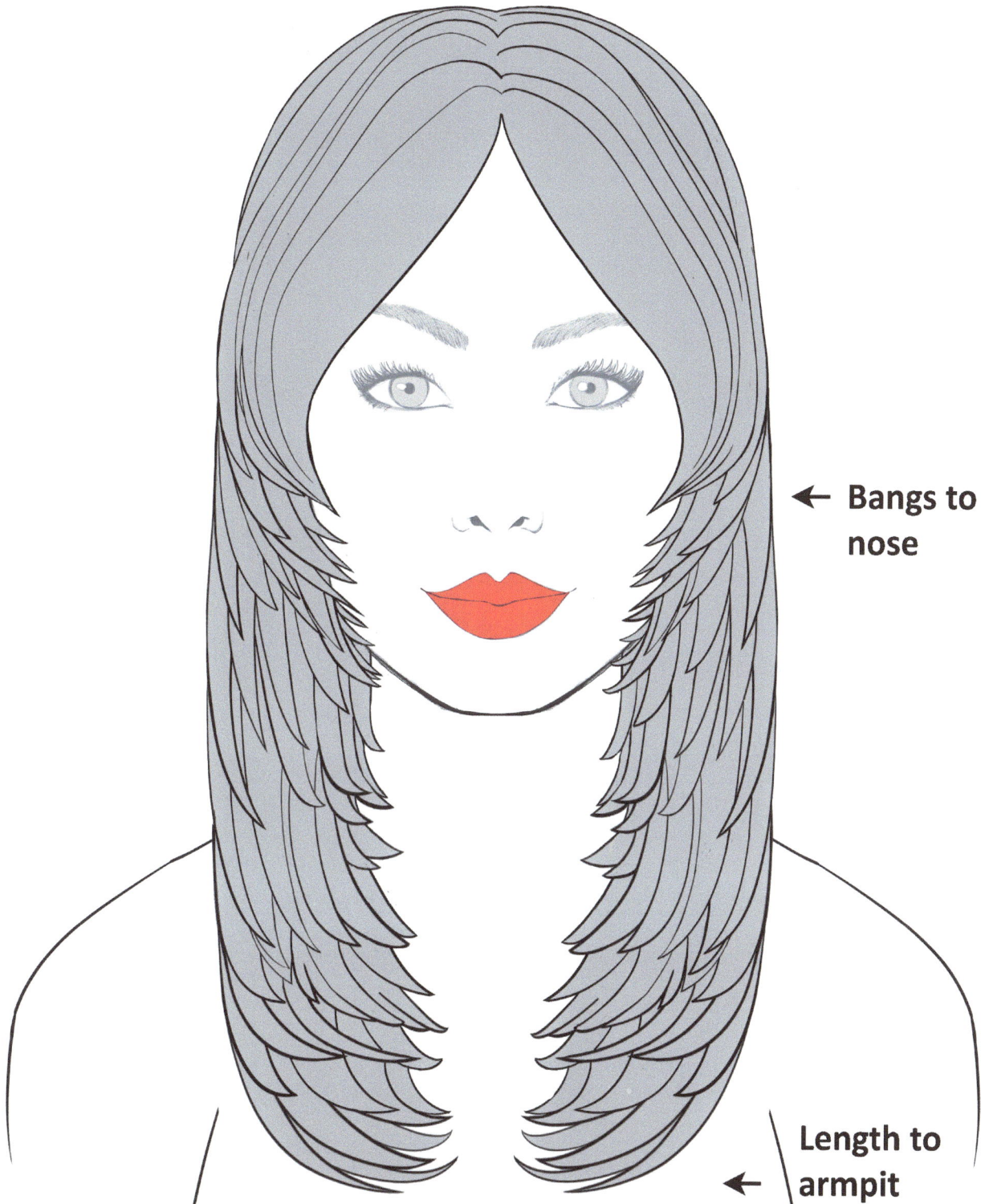

← **Bangs to nose**

← **Length to armpit**

LONG LENGTH - LONG BANGS

THE OVAL HAIRCUT

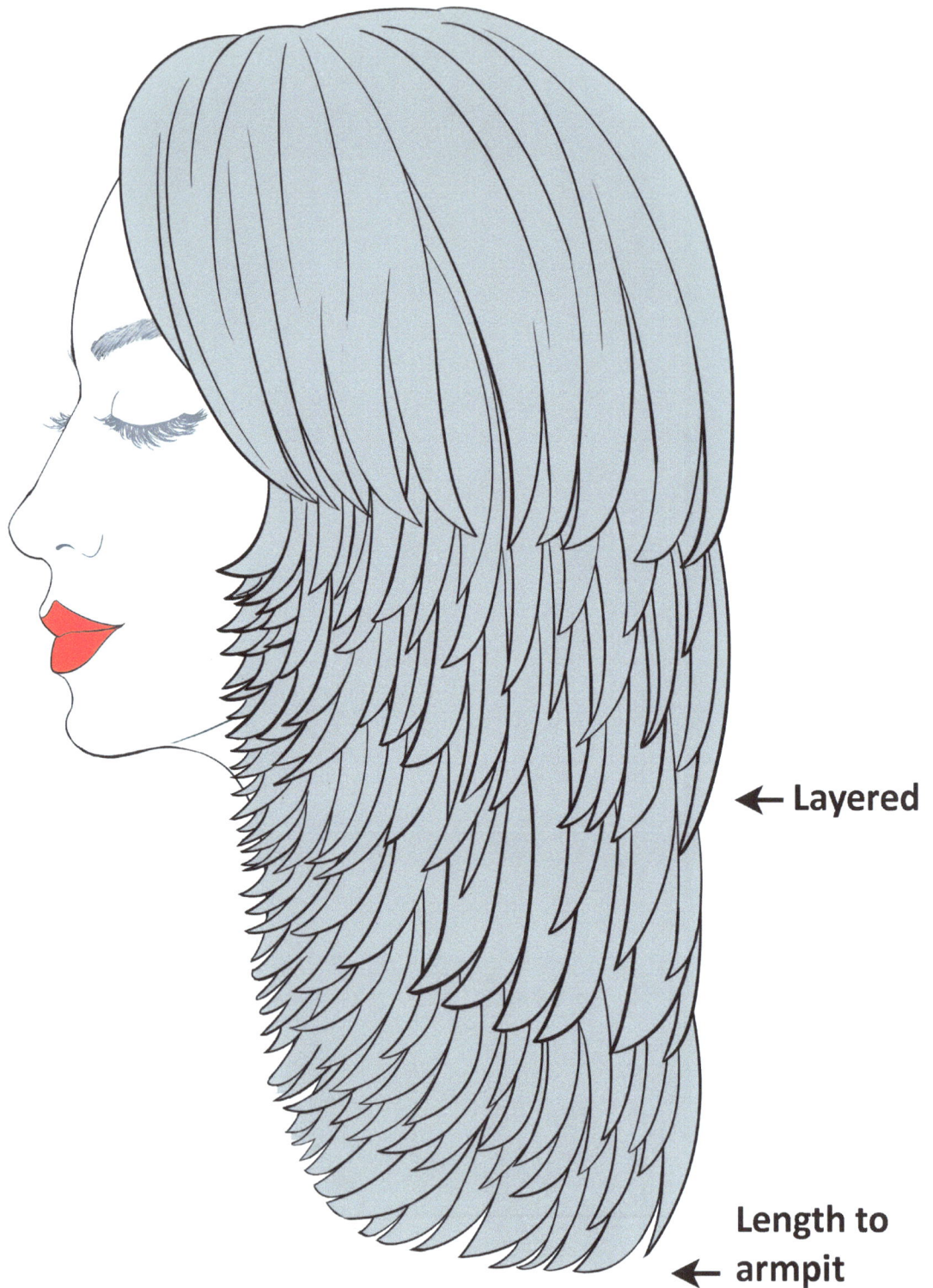

← Layered

Length to
← armpit

LONG LENGTH - LONG BANGS

THE OVAL HAIRCUT

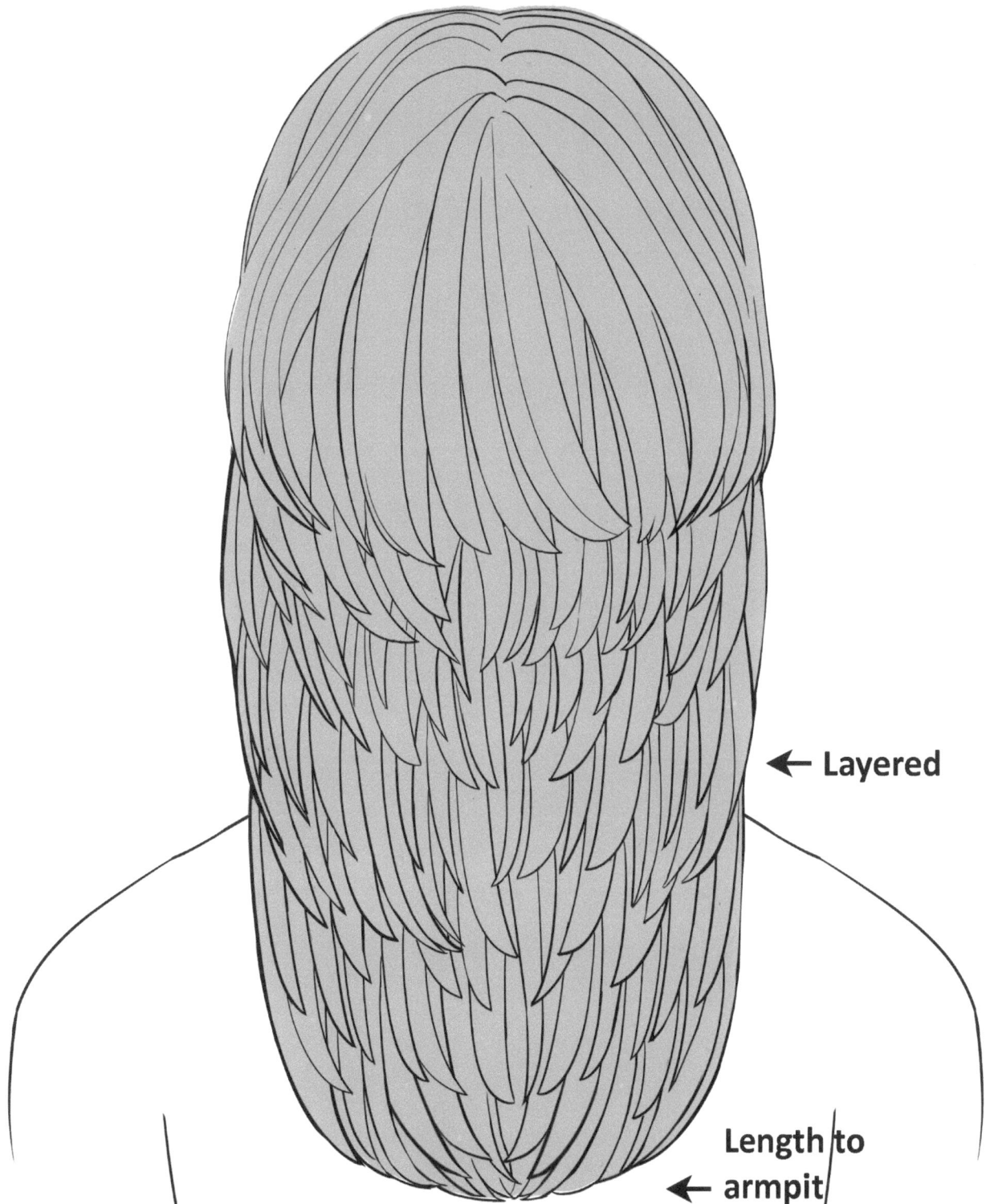

← Layered

Length to
← armpit

LONG LENGTH - LONG BANGS

THE OVAL HAIRCUT

Styling Options

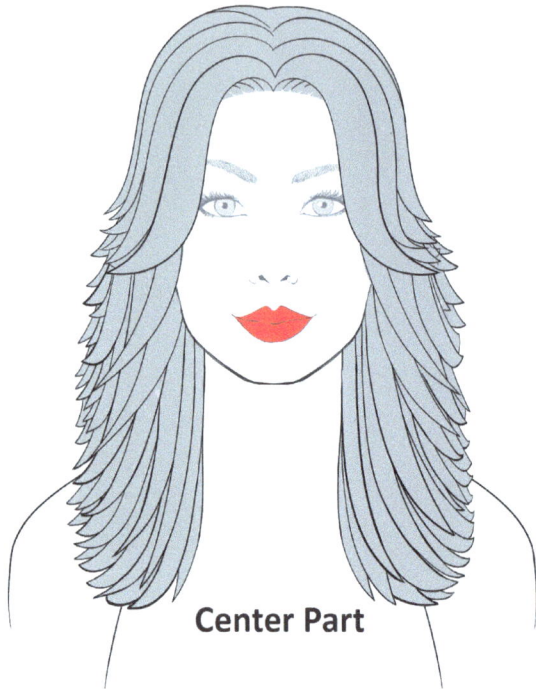

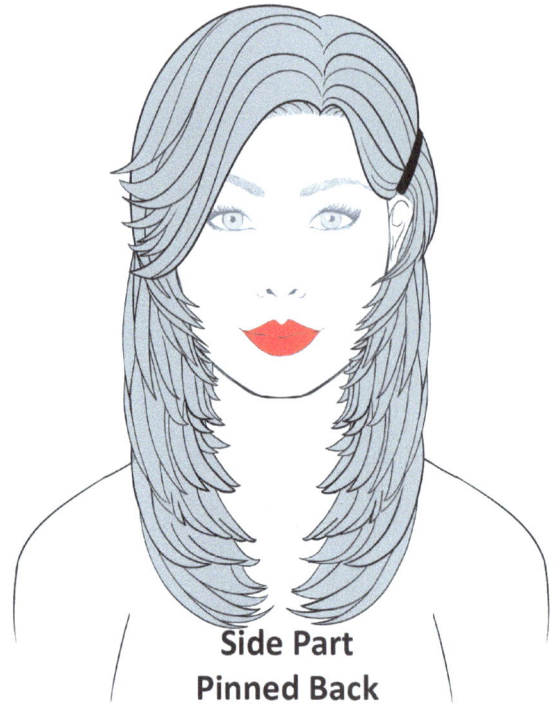

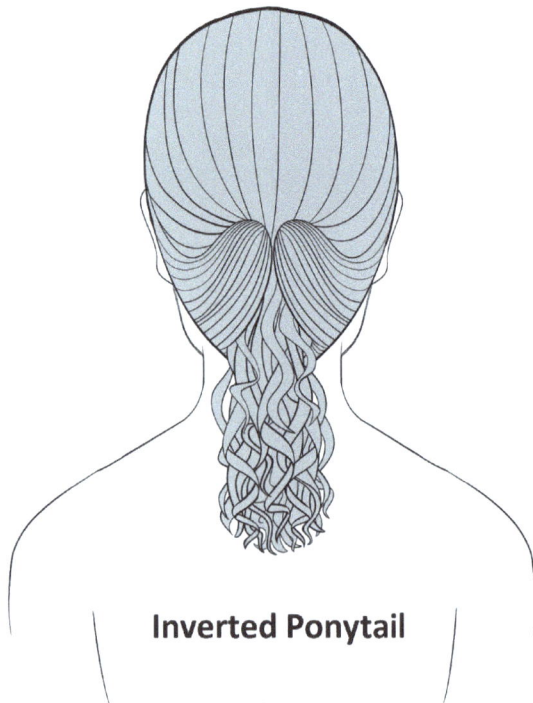

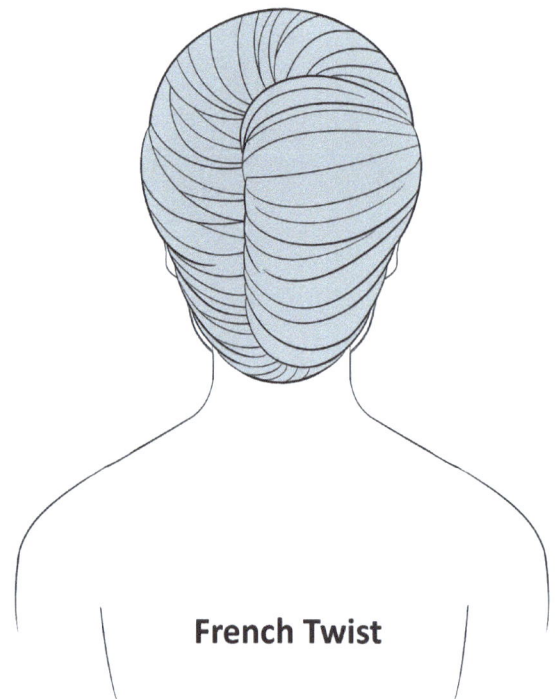

Center Part

**Side Part
Pinned Back**

Inverted Ponytail

French Twist

LONG LENGTH - LONG BANGS

THE OVAL HAIRCUT

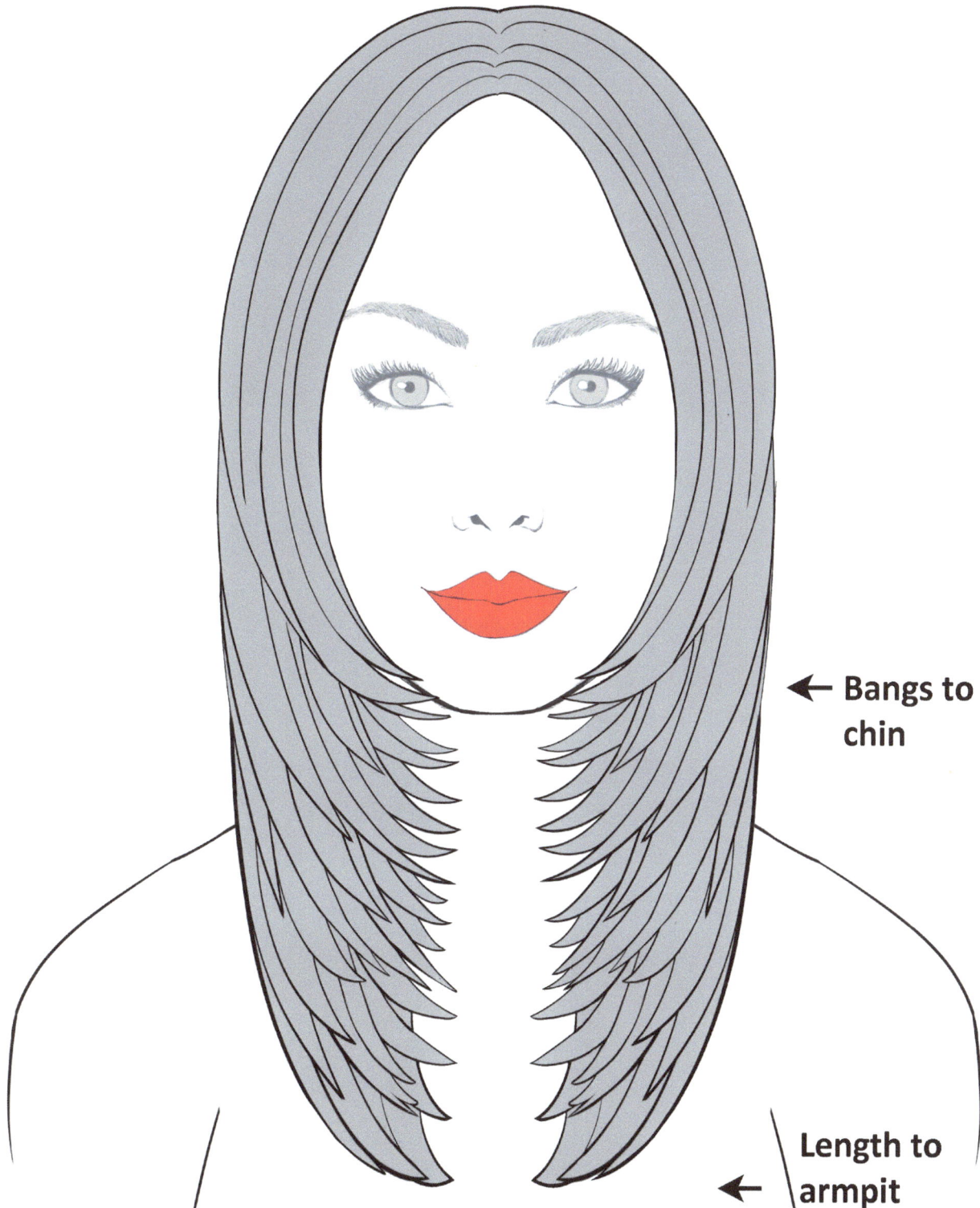

← **Bangs to chin**

← **Length to armpit**

LONG LENGTH - BANGS TO CHIN

THE OVAL HAIRCUT

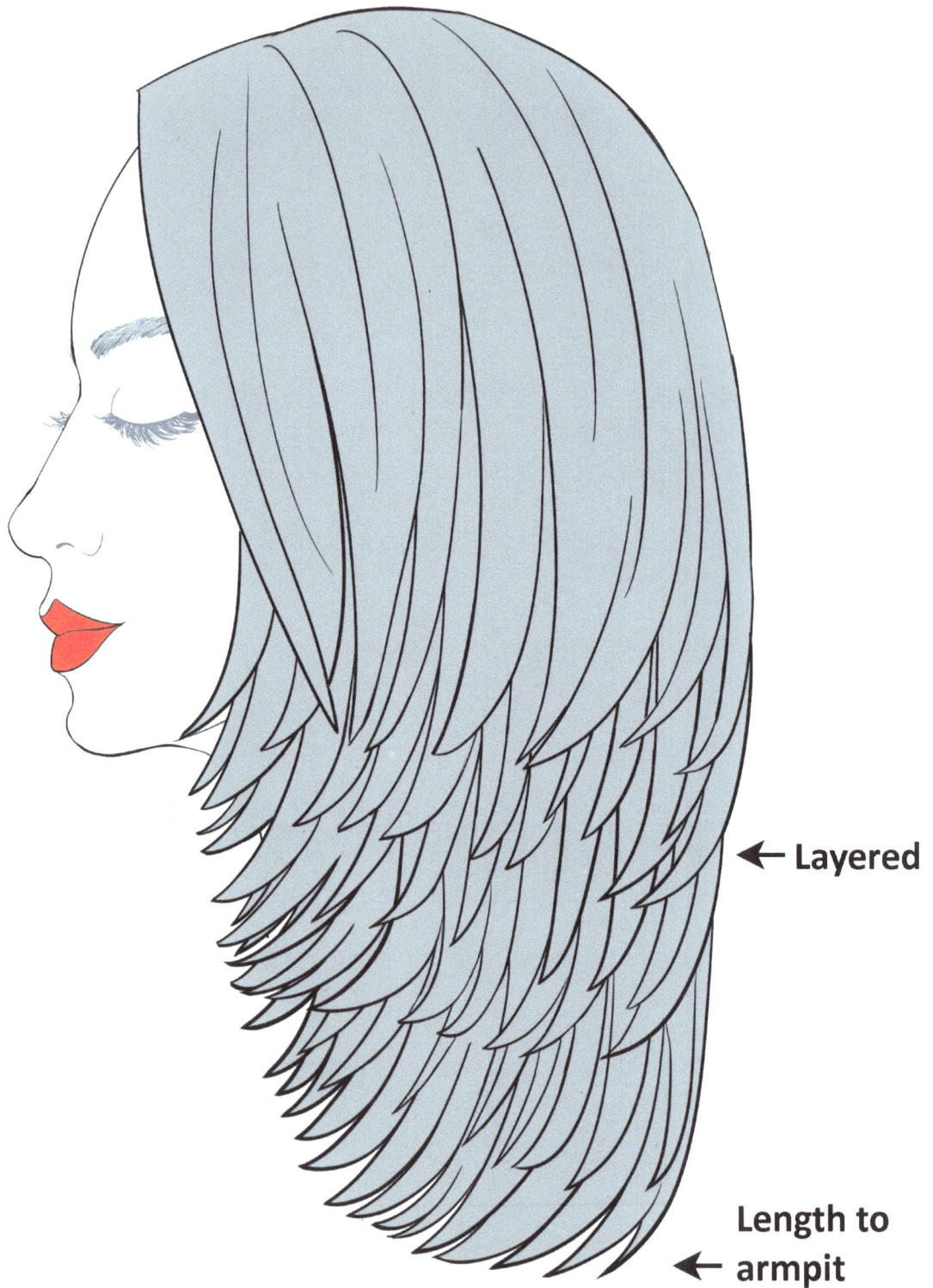

← Layered

Length to
← armpit

LONG LENGTH - BANGS TO CHIN

THE OVAL HAIRCUT

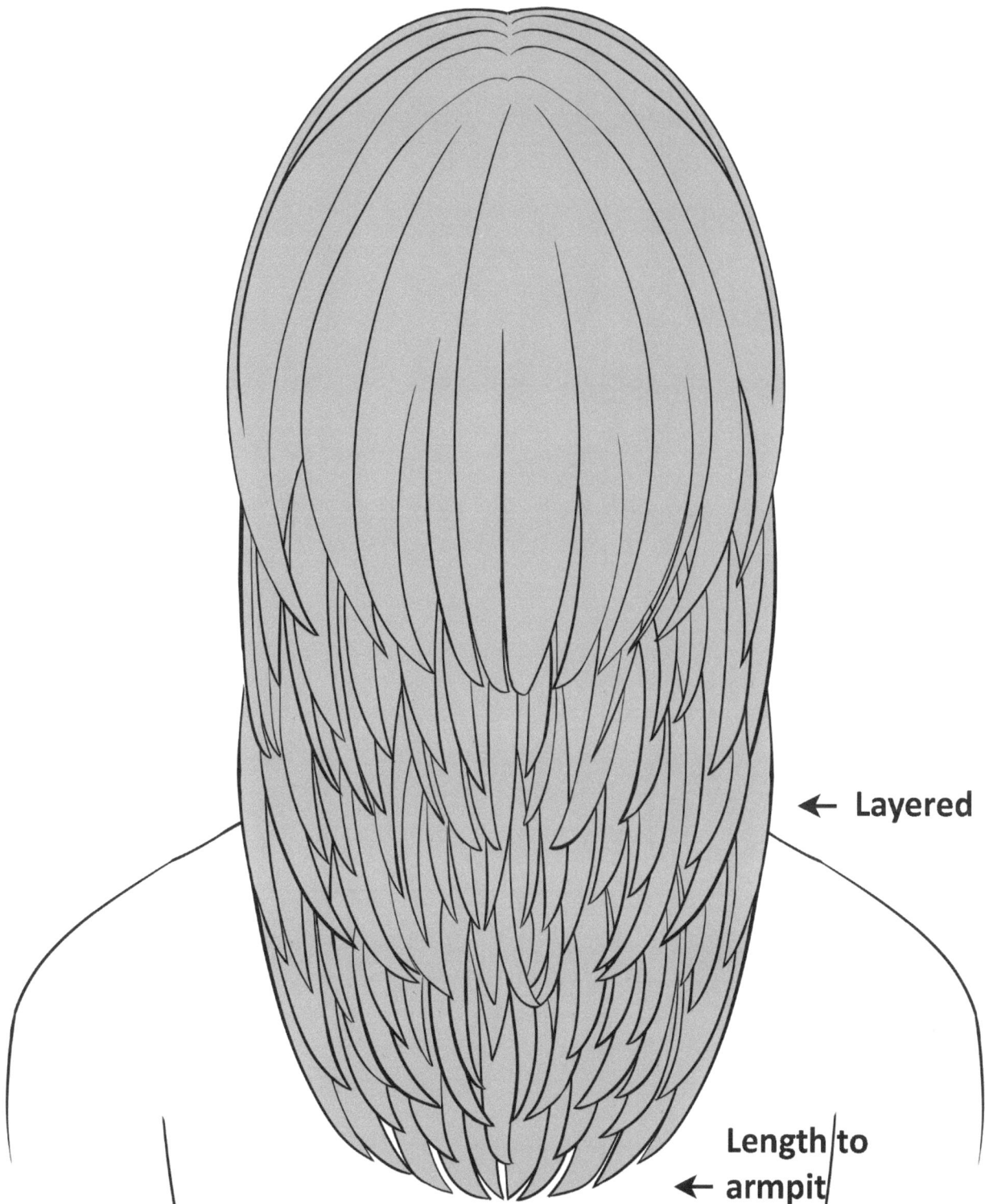

← Layered

Length to
← armpit

LONG LENGTH - BANGS TO CHIN

THE OVAL HAIRCUT

Styling Options

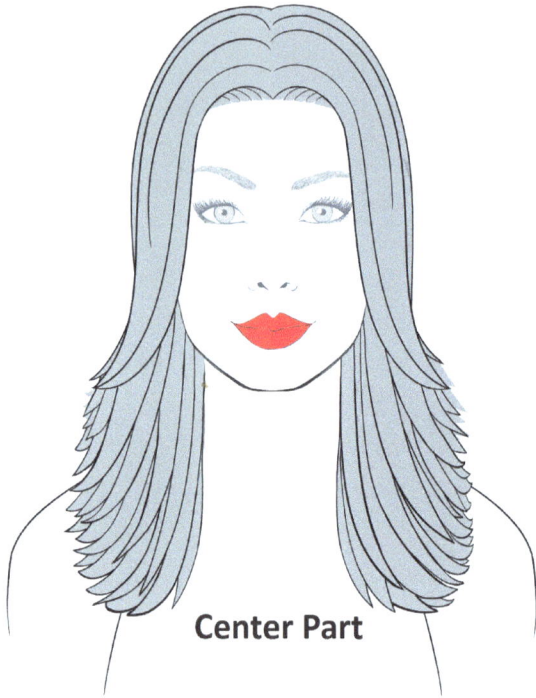

Center Part

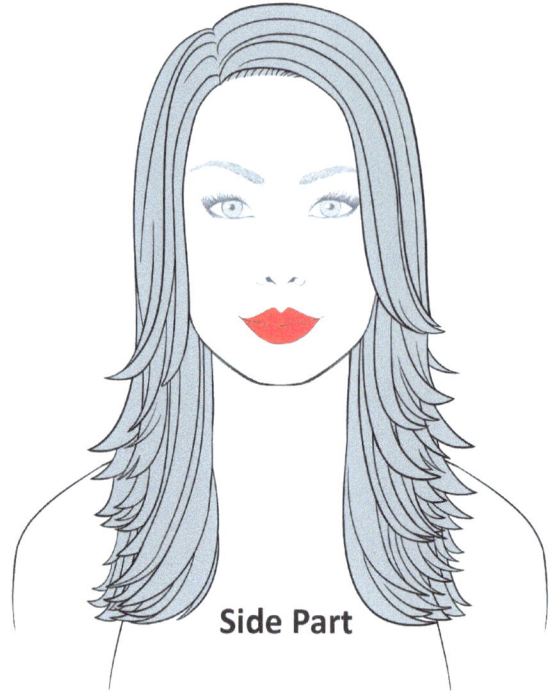

Side Part

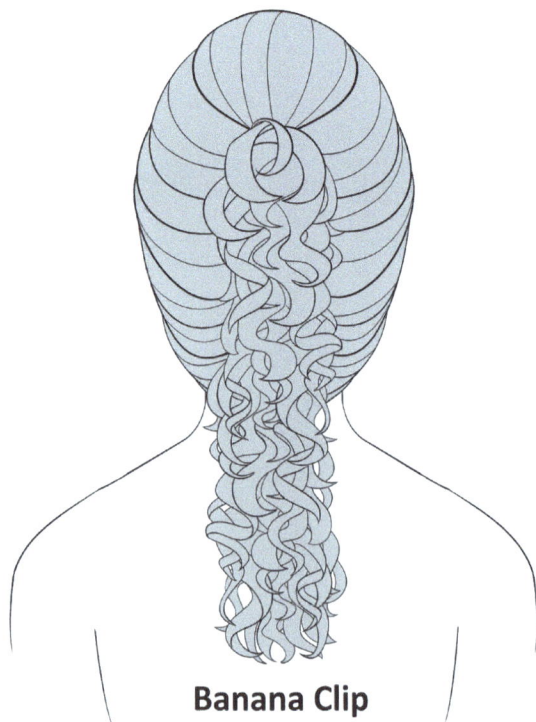

Banana Clip

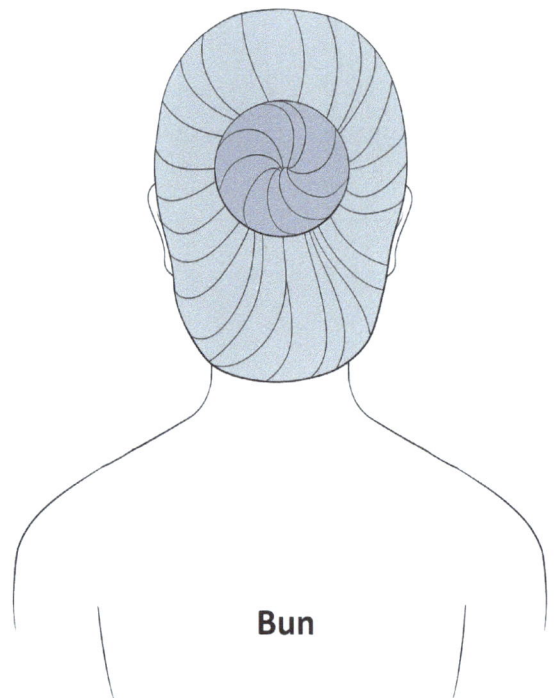

Bun

LONG LENGTH - BANGS TO CHIN

Chapter 2
THE ONE LENGTH HAIRCUT

This classic haircut offers dazzling beauty. Short and sassy or long and luscious, you decide.

- **LENGTH-** The One Length Haircut looks great in short lengths, medium lengths, and long lengths. Choose a round bottom or a straight bottom for the back length.

- **PART-** This haircut has a changeable part.

- **BANGS-** Looks great with or without bangs.

- **LAYERS-** There are no layers in a One Length Haircut.

- **STYLING-** The One Length Haircut has many styling options. Style your hair straight or curled, up or down, and every way in between. Longer lengths look great in updo's, ponytails and braids.

THE ONE LENGTH HAIRCUT

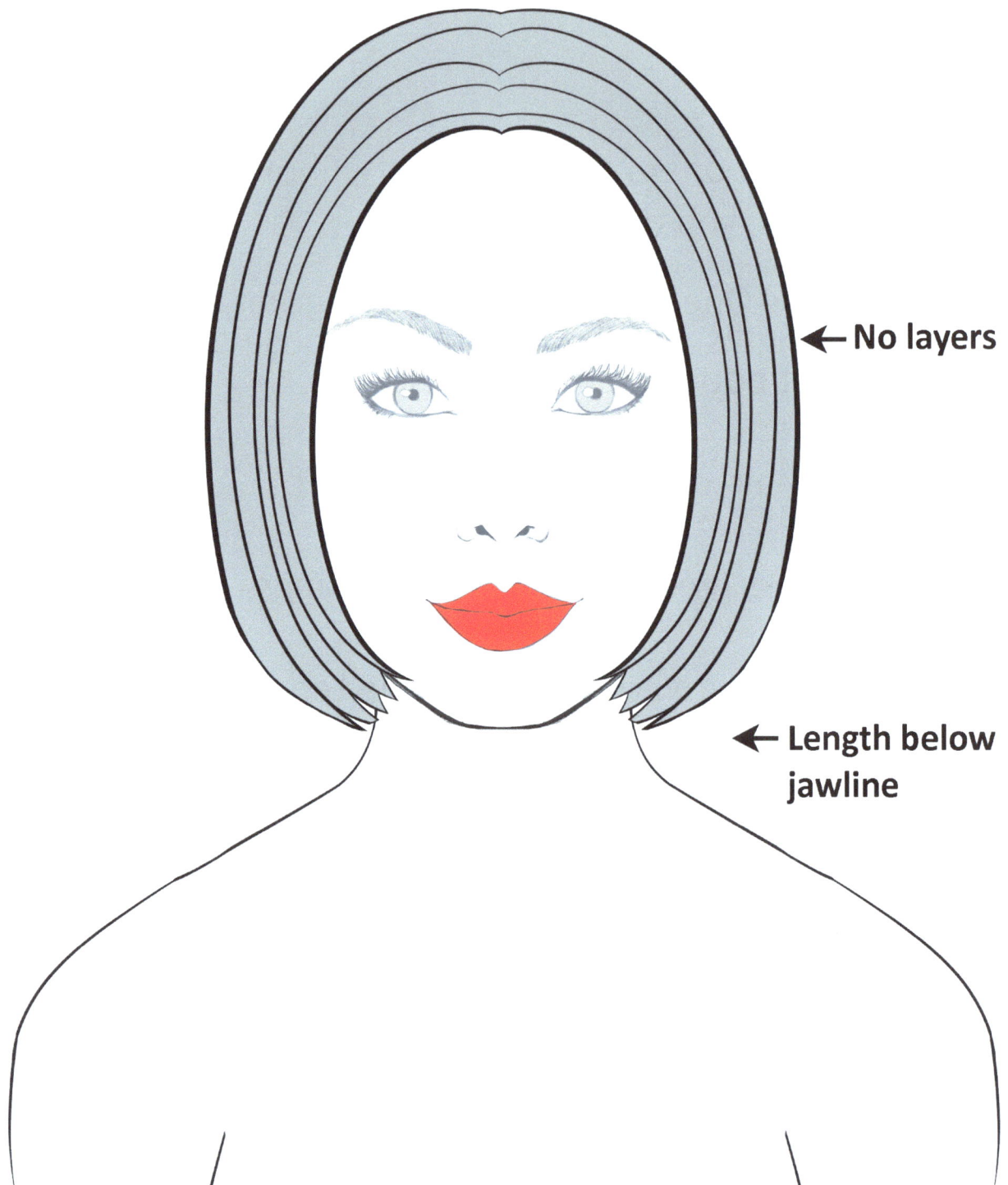

← No layers

← Length below
jawline

SHORT LENGTH - ROUND BOTTOM

THE ONE LENGTH HAIRCUT

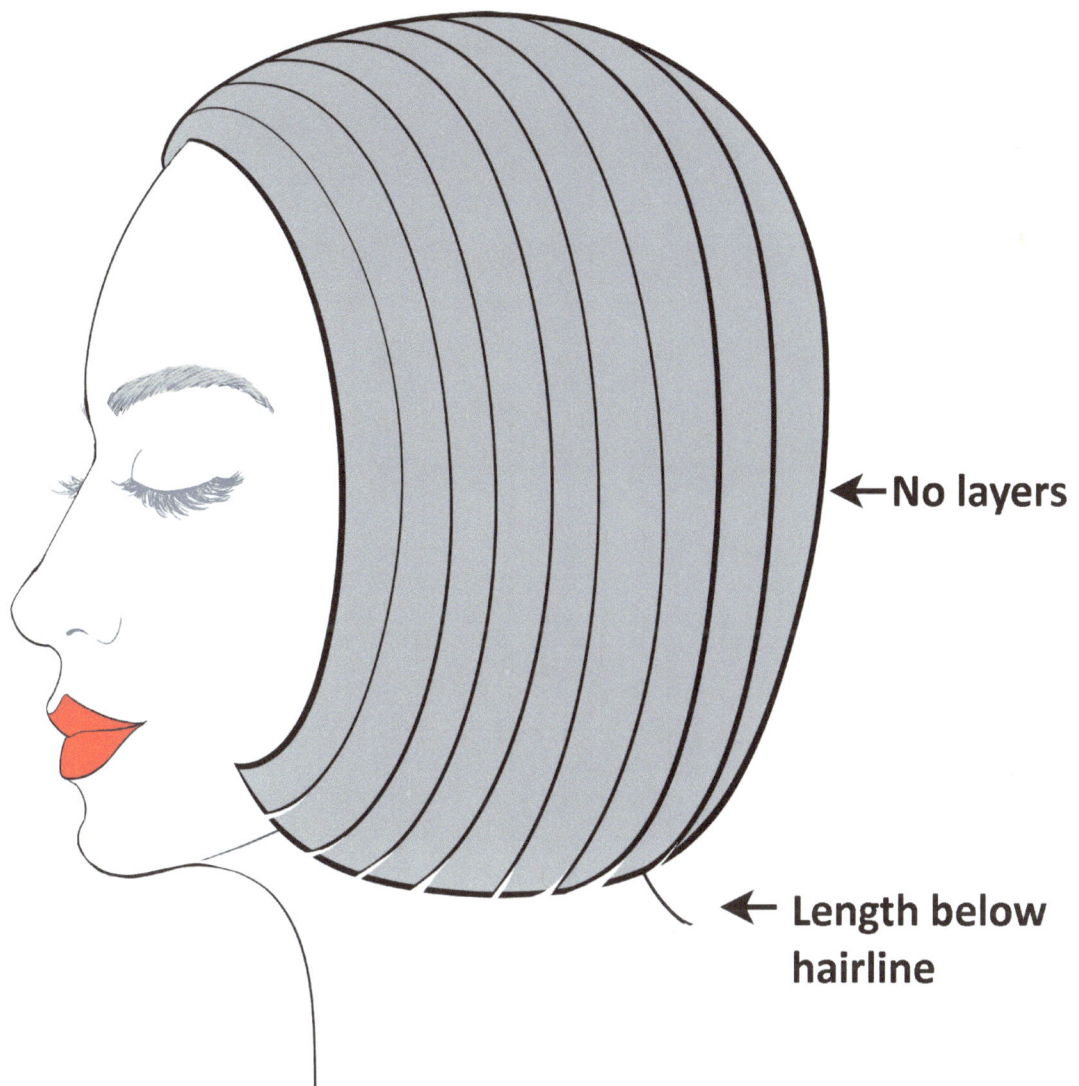

← **No layers**

← **Length below hairline**

SHORT LENGTH - ROUND BOTTOM

THE ONE LENGTH HAIRCUT

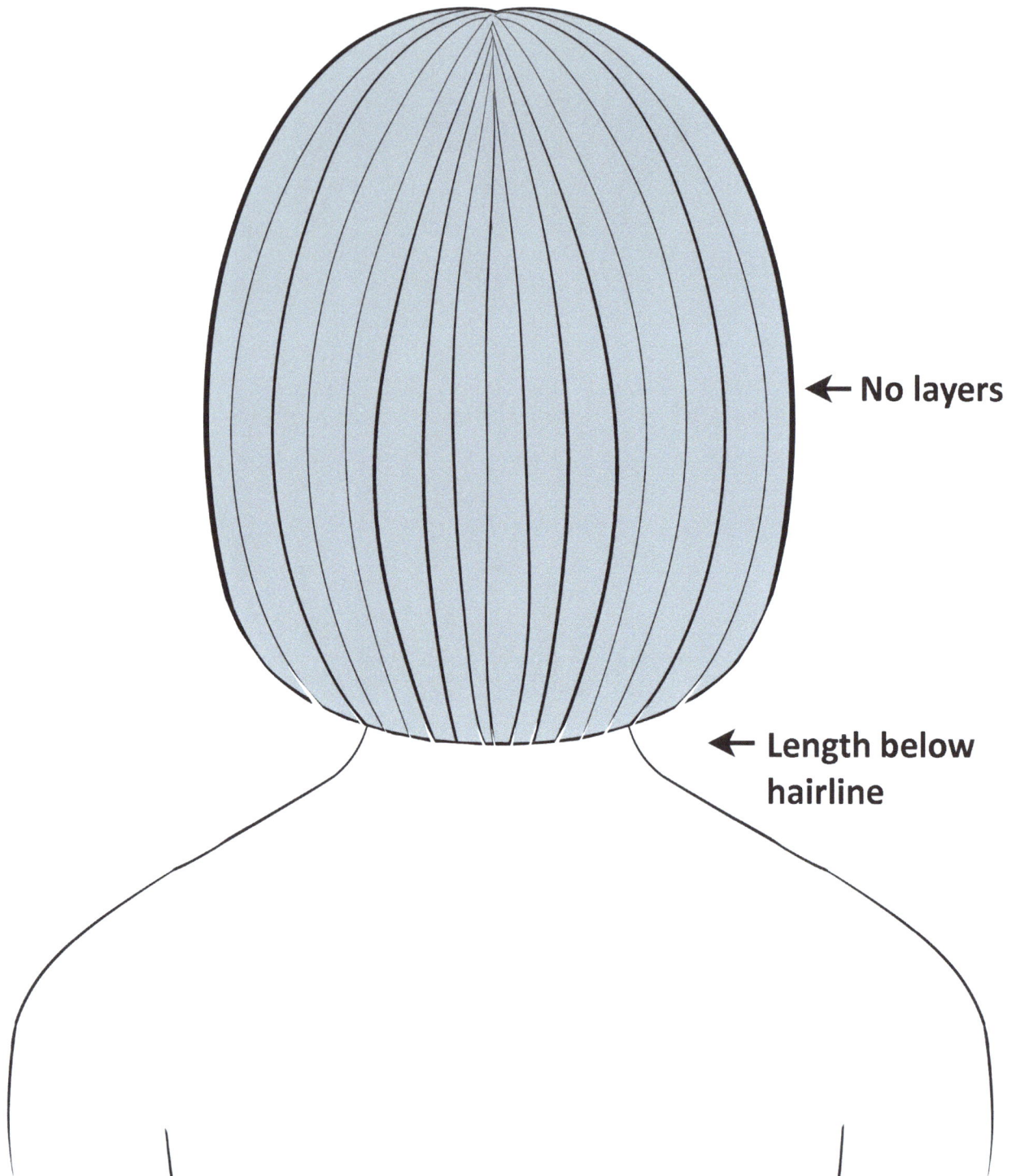

← **No layers**

← **Length below hairline**

SHORT LENGTH - ROUND BOTTOM

THE ONE LENGTH HAIRCUT

Styling Options

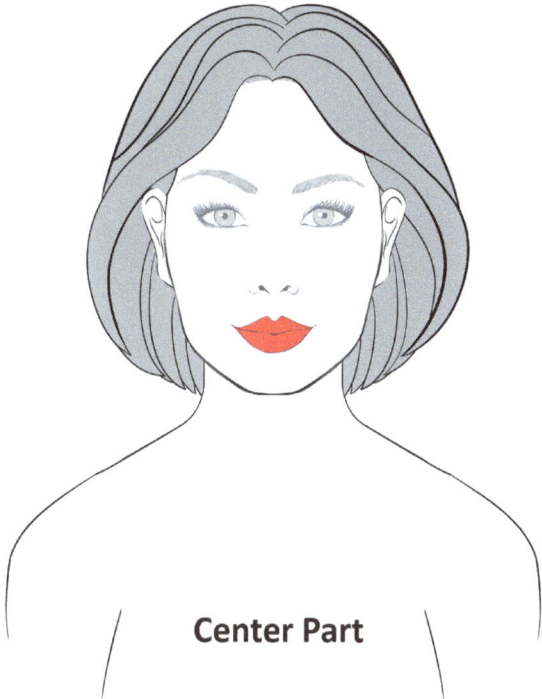

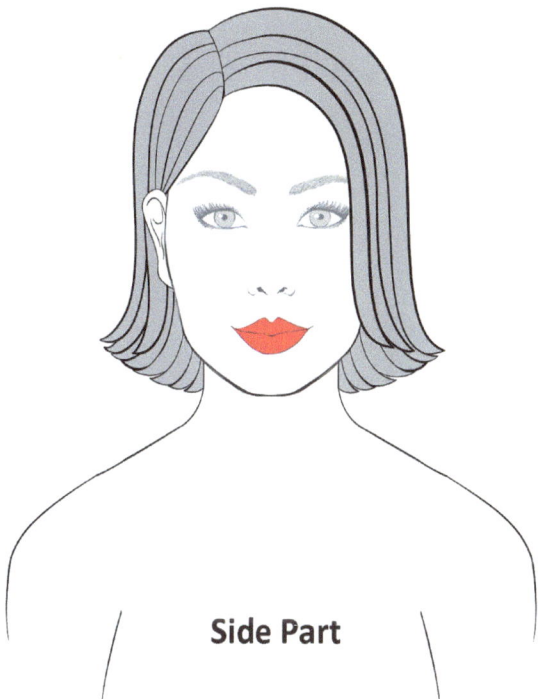

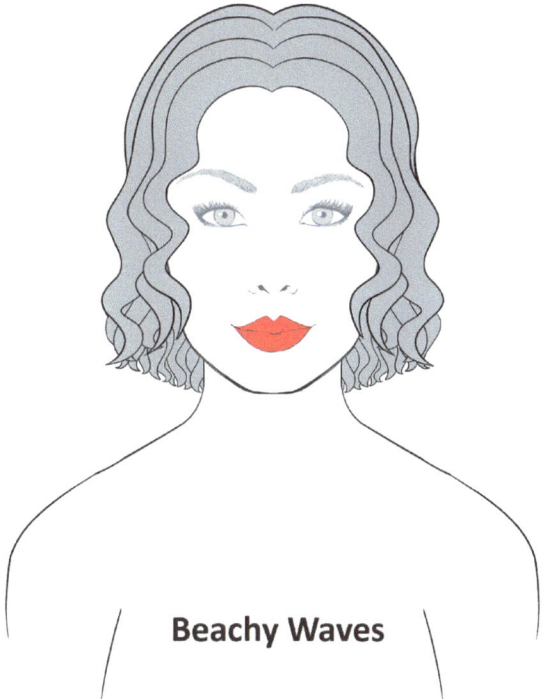

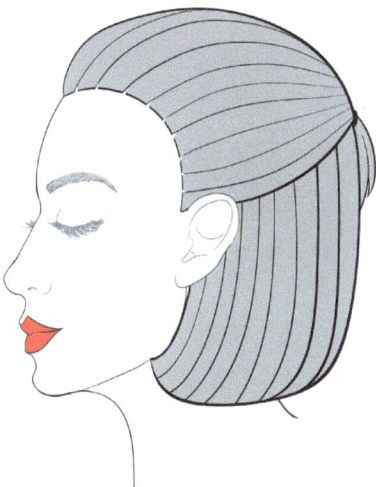

Center Part

Side Part

Beachy Waves

Half Up-Do

SHORT LENGTH - ROUND BOTTOM

THE ONE LENGTH HAIRCUT

Styling Options with Bangs

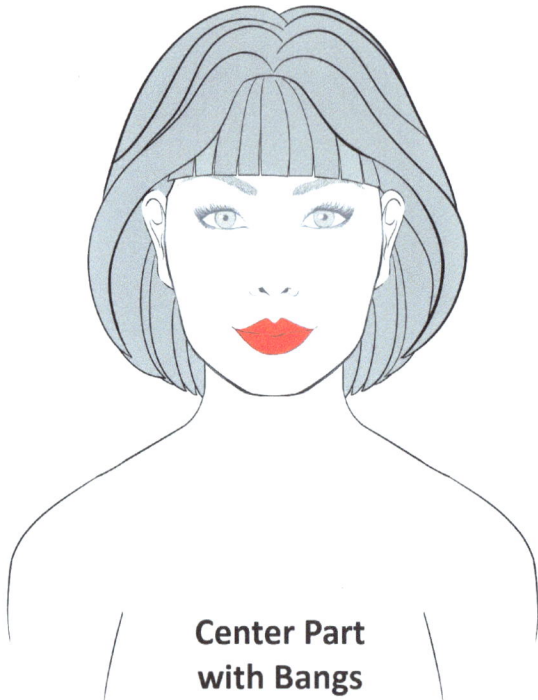

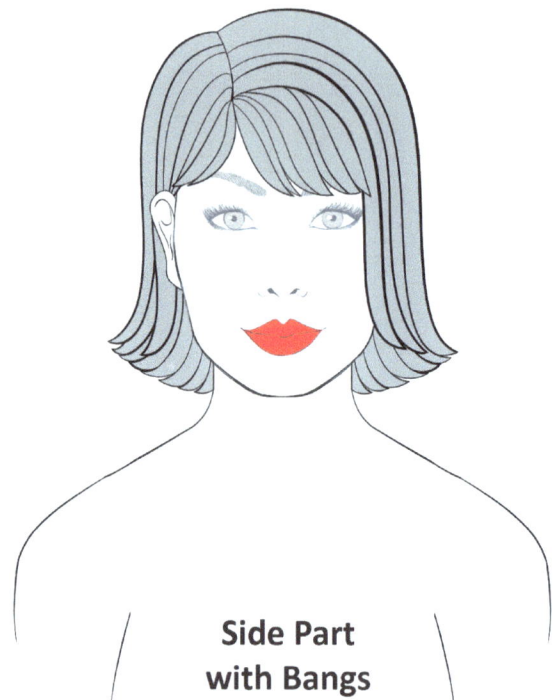

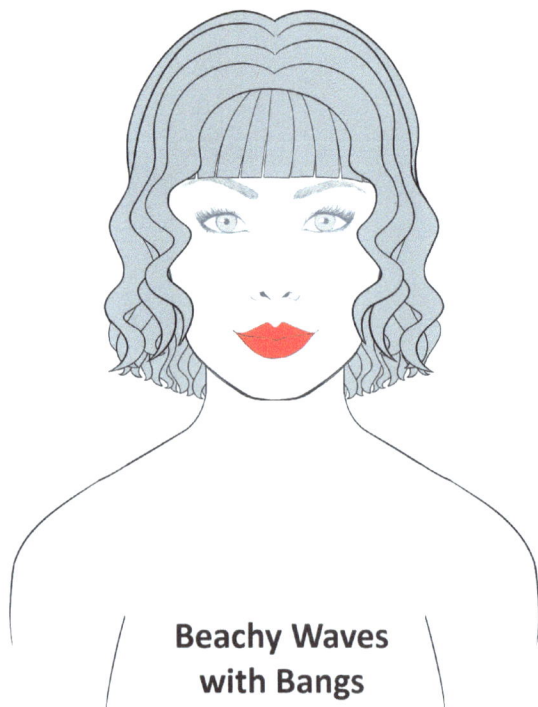

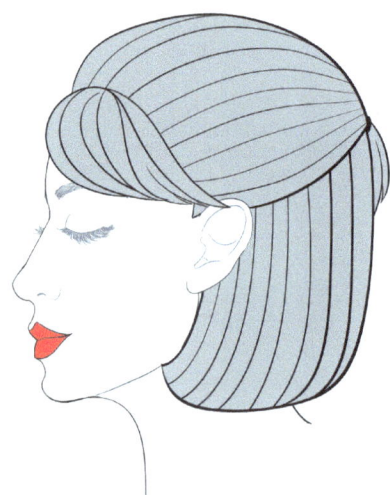

**Center Part
with Bangs**

**Side Part
with Bangs**

**Beachy Waves
with Bangs**

**Half Up-Do
with Bangs**

SHORT LENGTH - ROUND BOTTOM

THE ONE LENGTH HAIRCUT

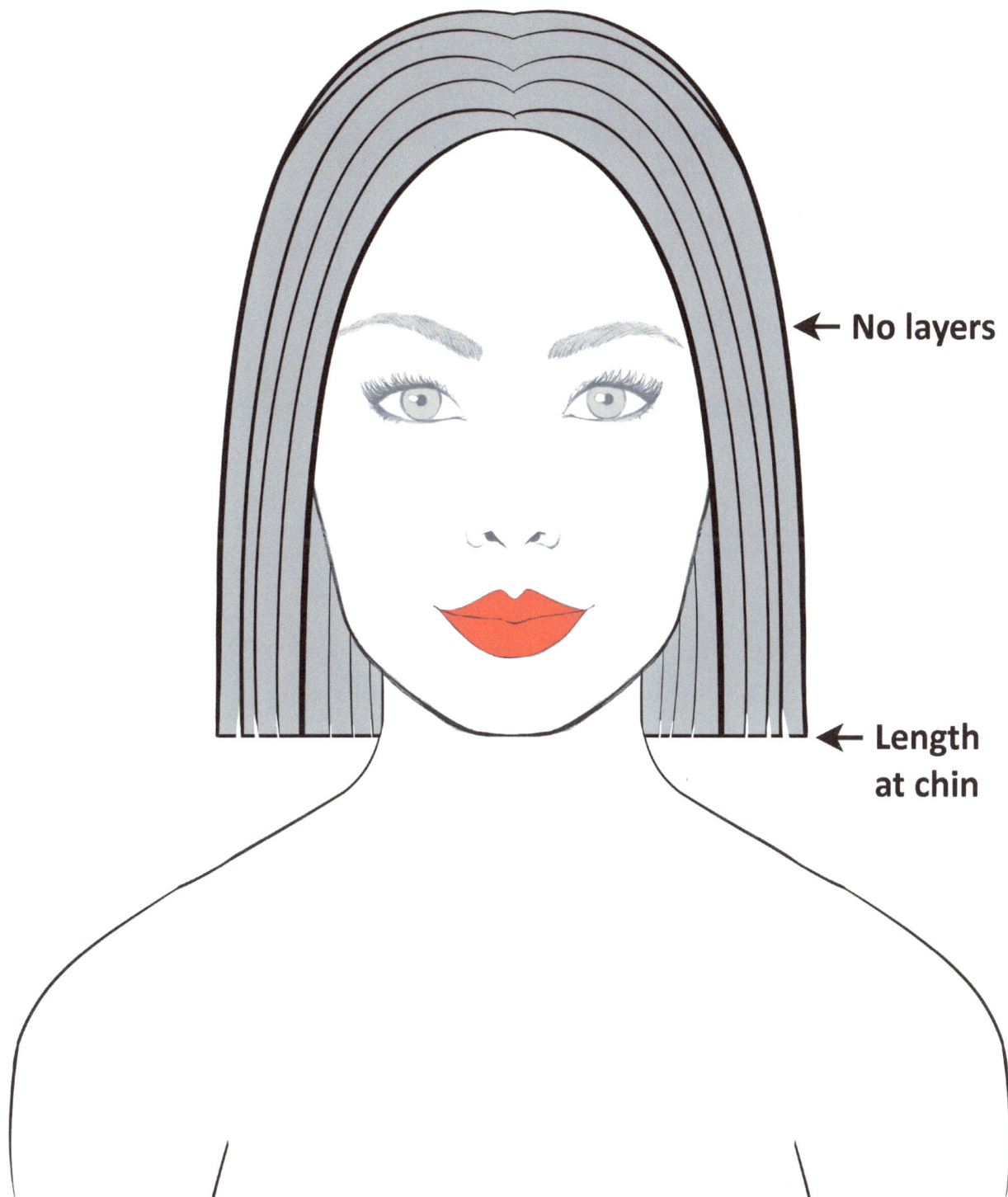

← No layers

← Length at chin

SHORT LENGTH - STRAIGHT BOTTOM

THE ONE LENGTH HAIRCUT

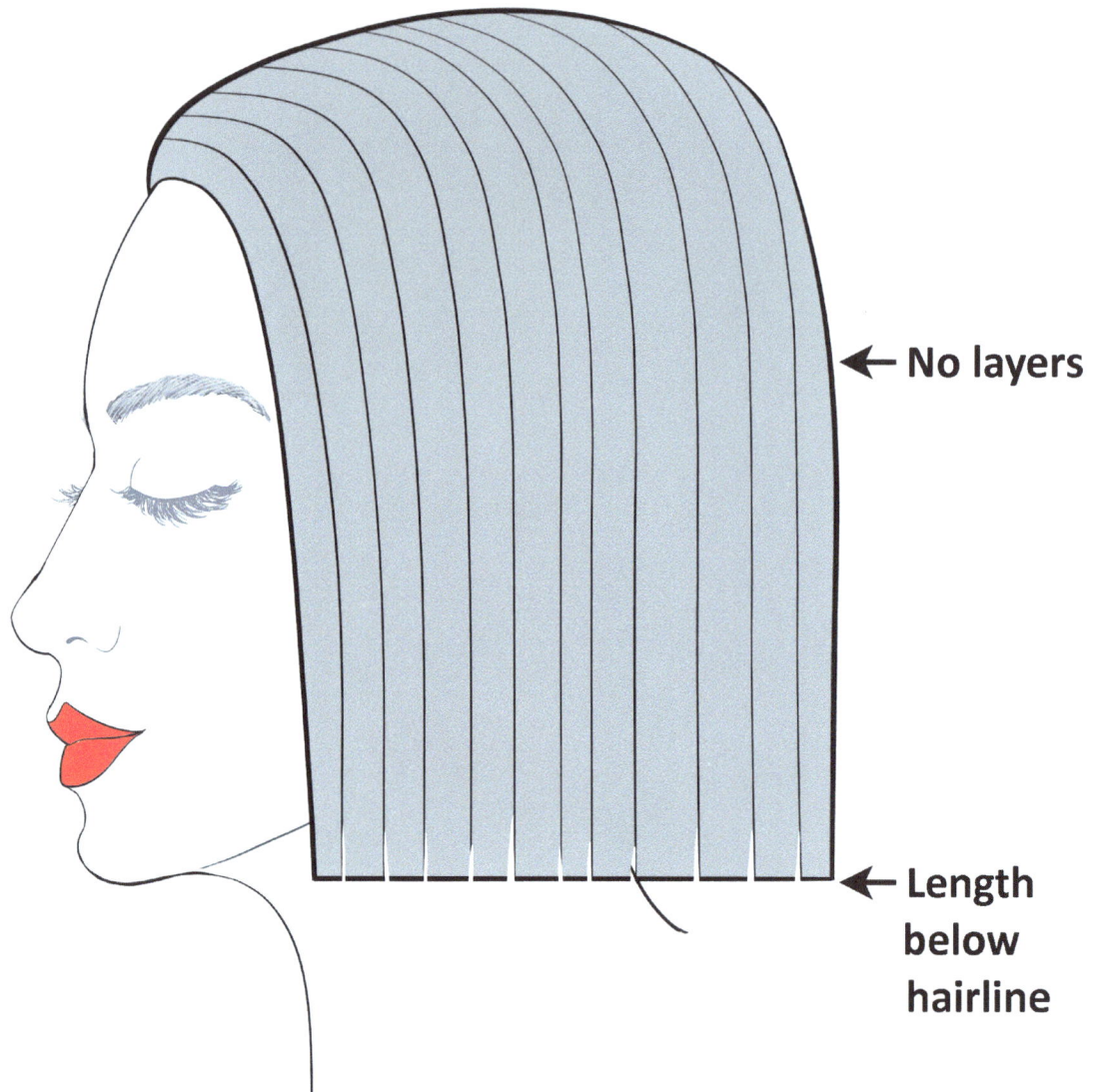

← No layers

← Length below hairline

SHORT LENGTH - STRAIGHT BOTTOM

THE ONE LENGTH HAIRCUT

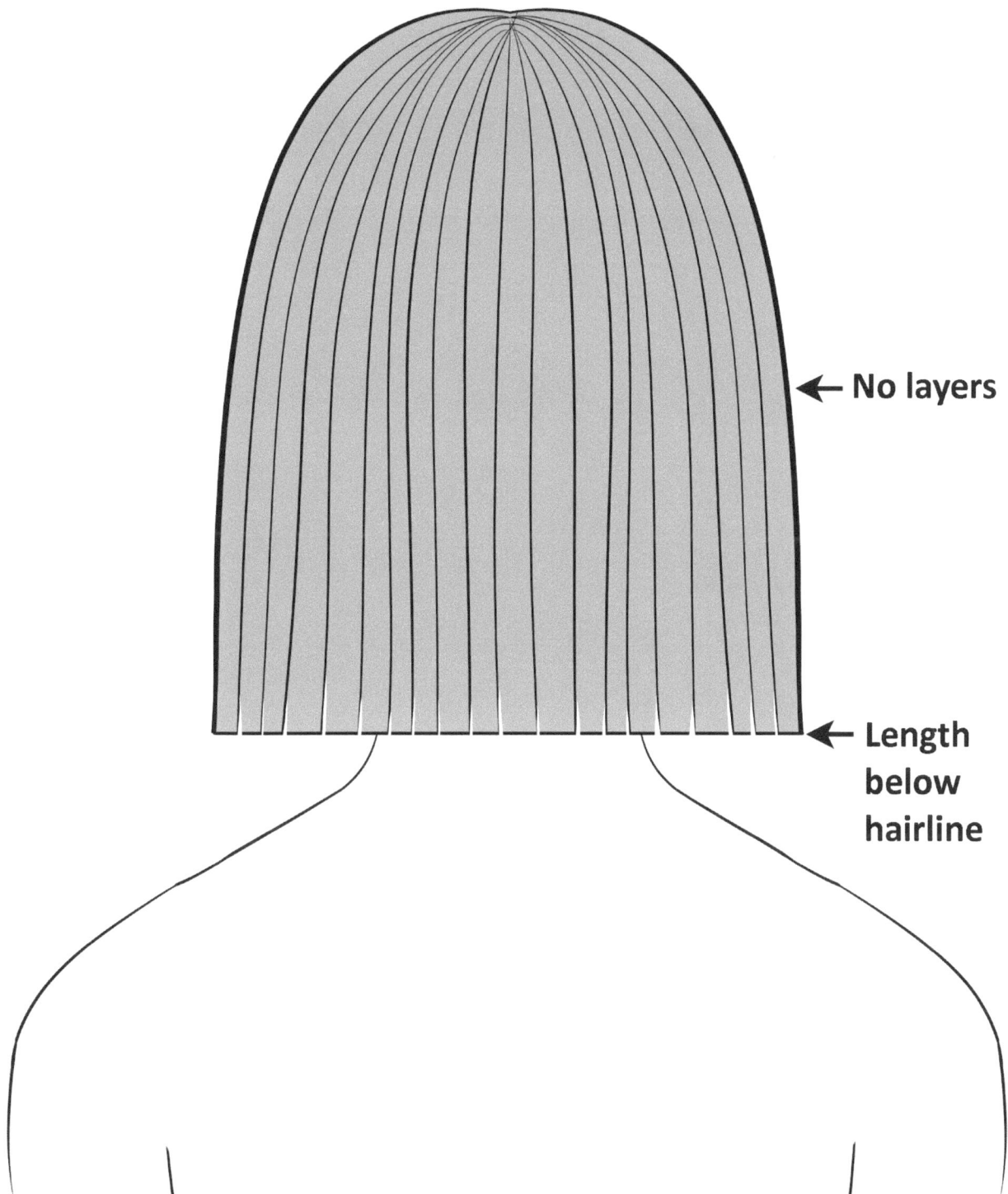

← No layers

← Length below hairline

SHORT LENGTH - STRAIGHT BOTTOM

THE ONE LENGTH HAIRCUT

Styling Options

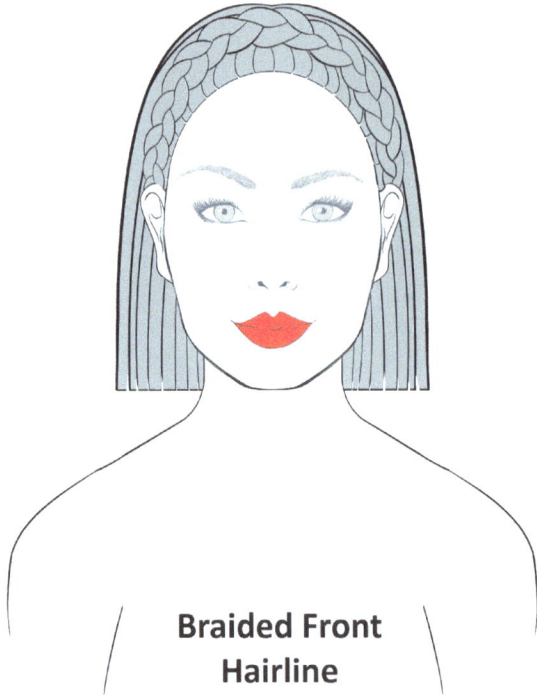

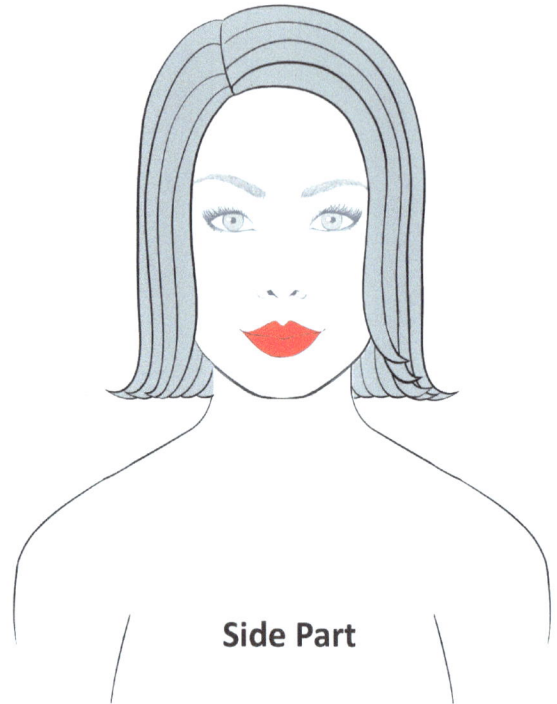

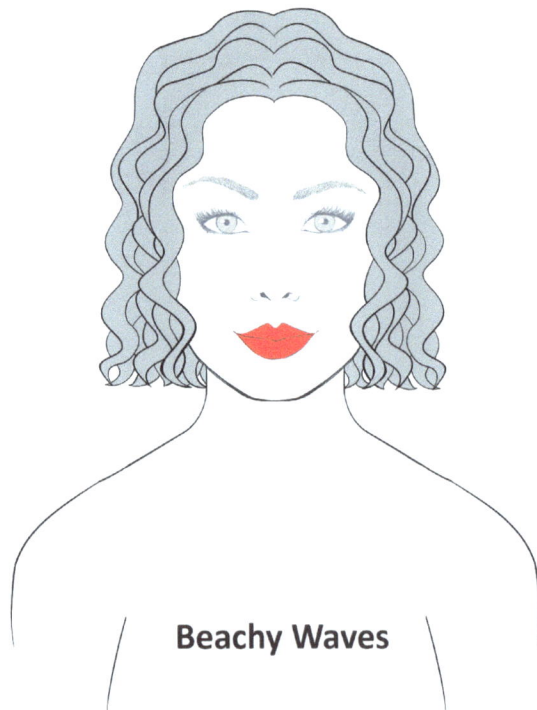

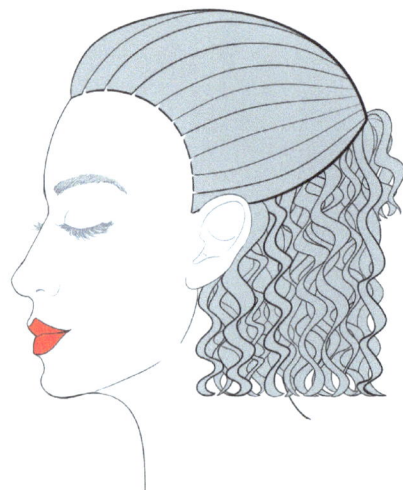

Braided Front Hairline

Side Part

Beachy Waves

Half Up-Do

SHORT LENGTH - STRAIGHT BOTTOM

THE ONE LENGTH HAIRCUT

Styling Options with Bangs

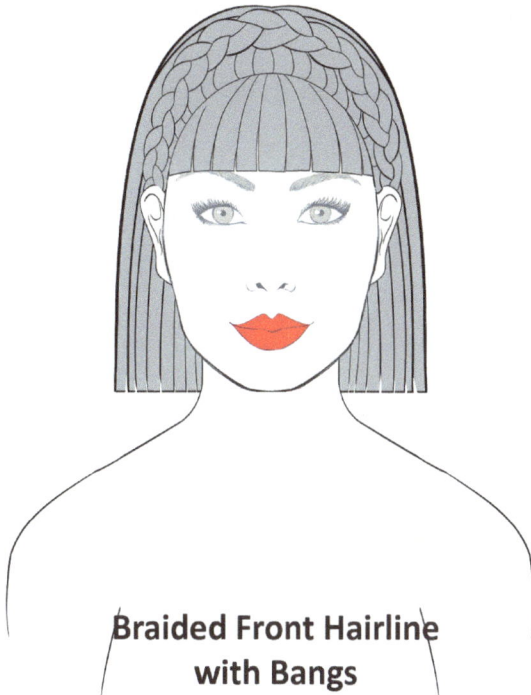

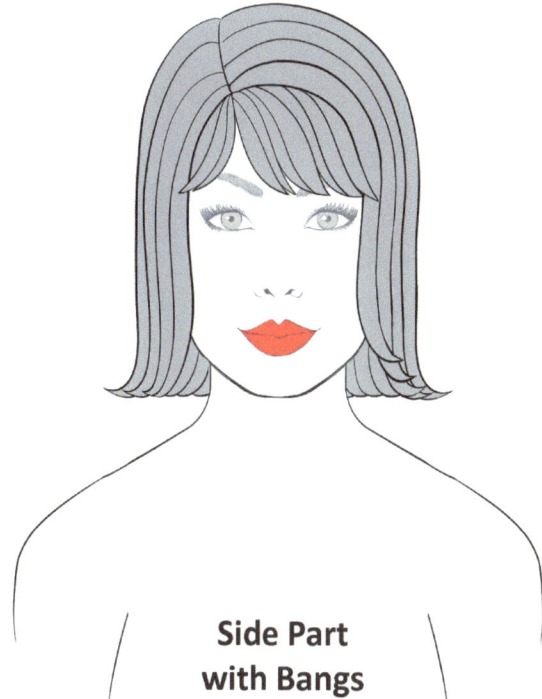

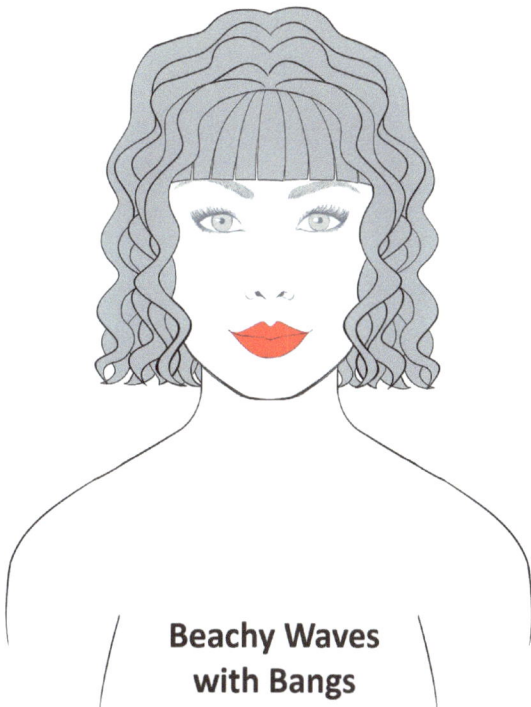

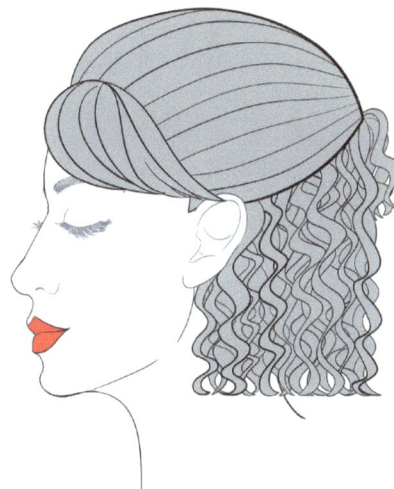

**Braided Front Hairline
with Bangs**

**Side Part
with Bangs**

**Beachy Waves
with Bangs**

**Half Up-Do
with Bangs**

SHORT LENGTH - STRAIGHT BOTTOM

THE ONE LENGTH HAIRCUT

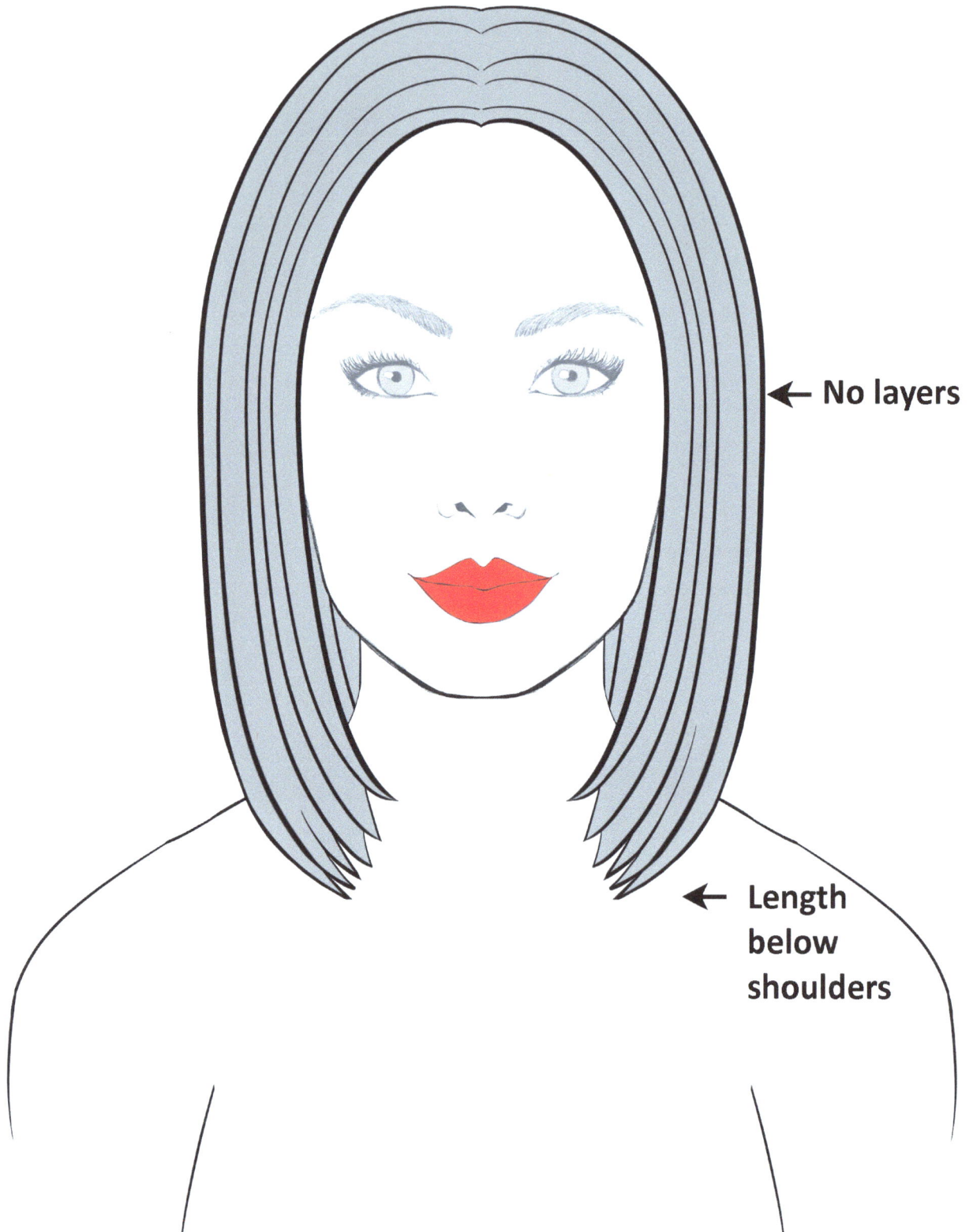

← No layers

← Length below shoulders

MEDIUM LENGTH - ROUND BOTTOM

THE ONE LENGTH HAIRCUT

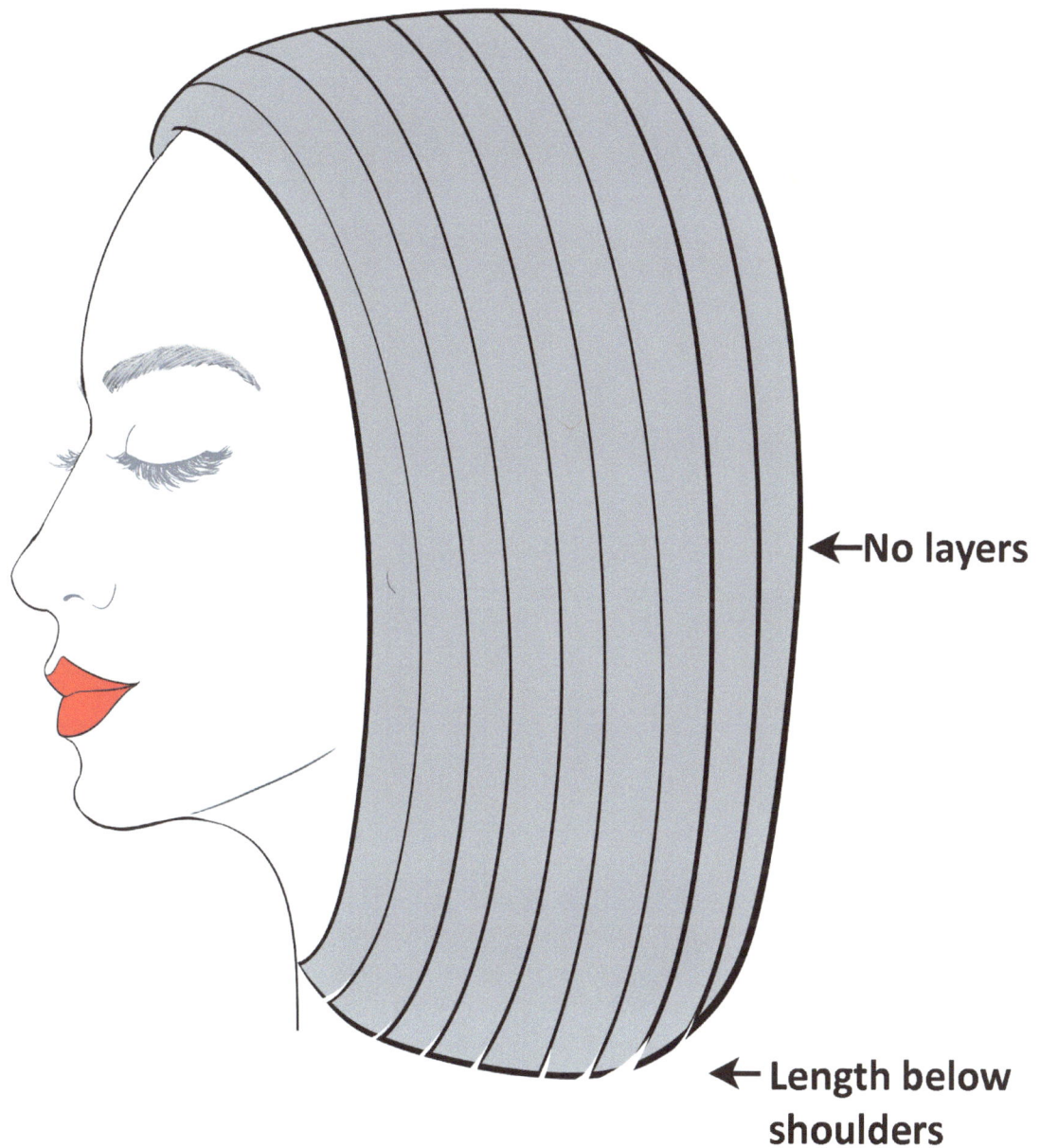

←No layers

← Length below
shoulders

MEDIUM LENGTH - ROUND BOTTOM

THE ONE LENGTH HAIRCUT

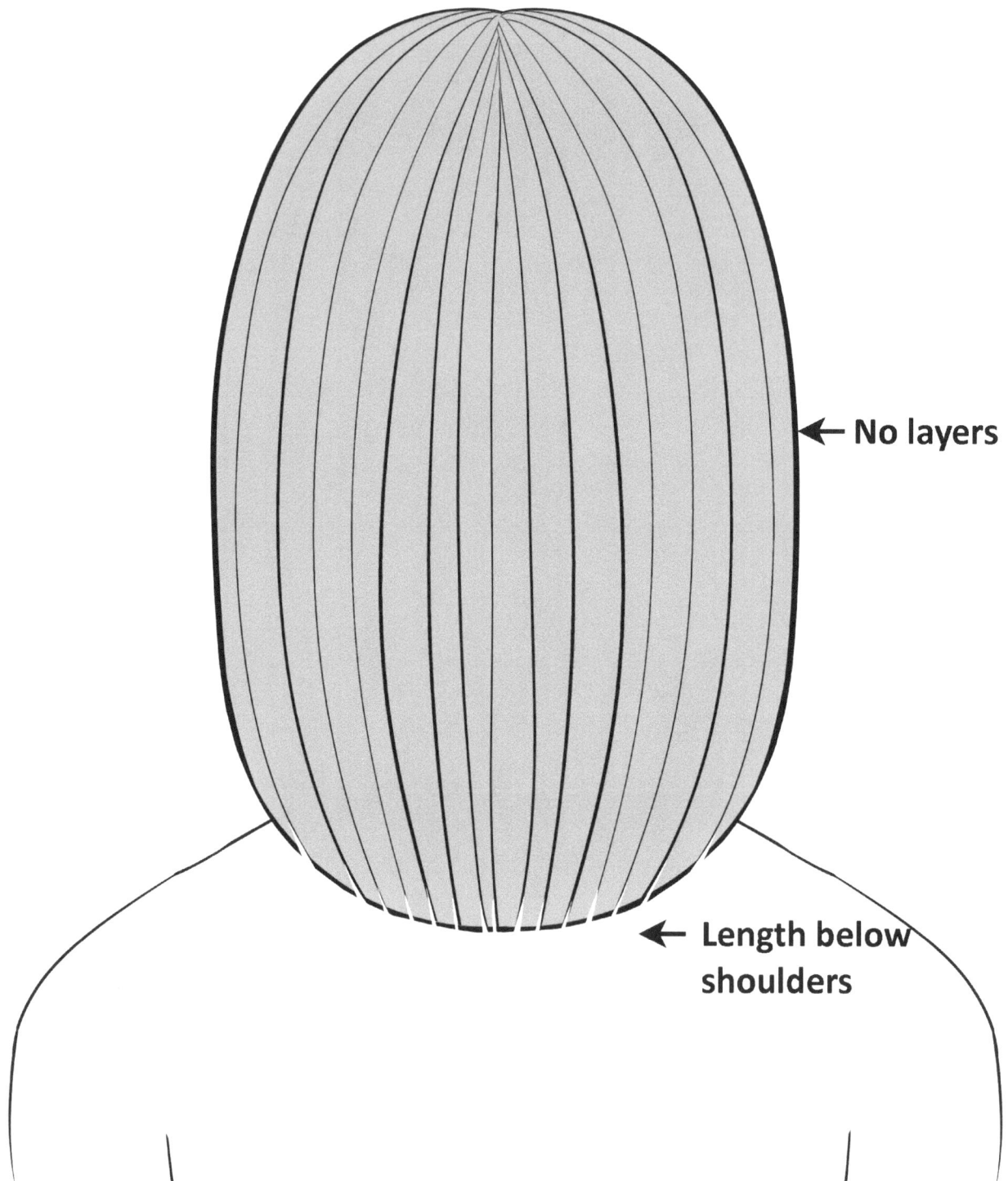

← No layers

← Length below
shoulders

MEDIUM LENGTH - ROUND BOTTOM

THE ONE LENGTH HAIRCUT

Styling Options

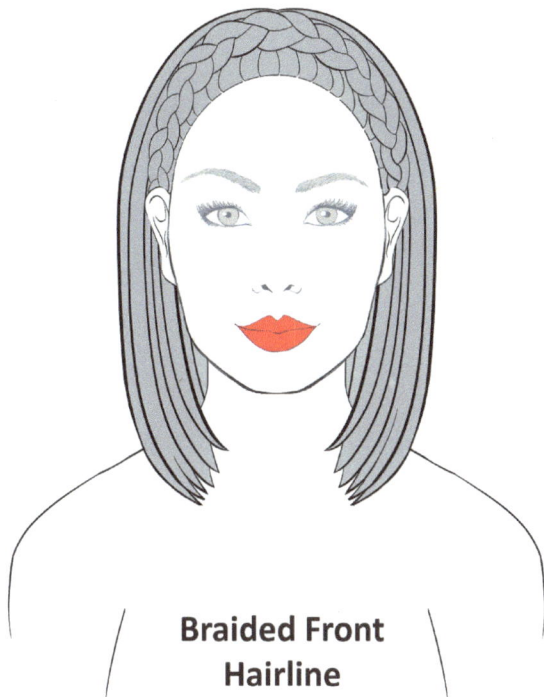

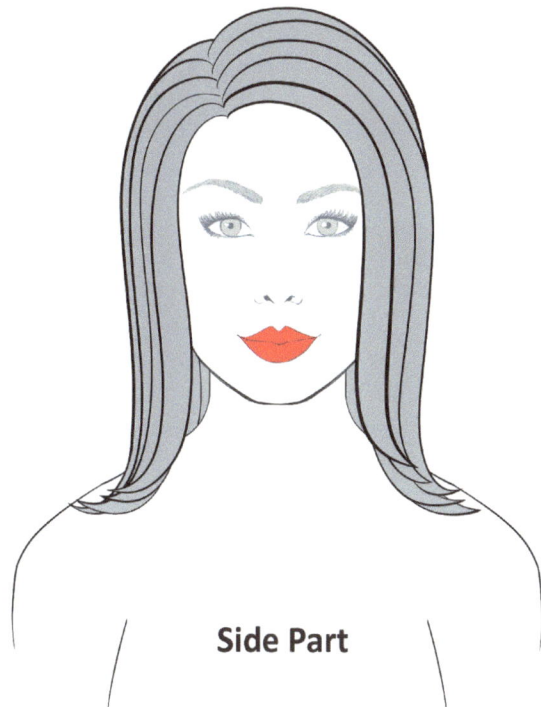

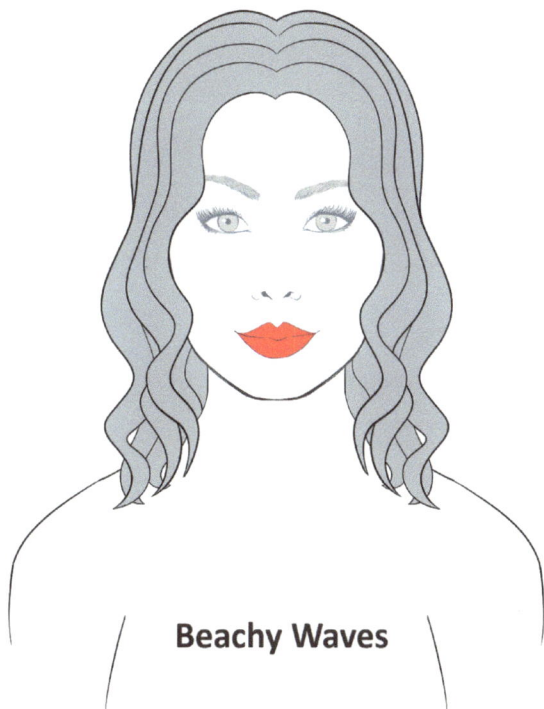

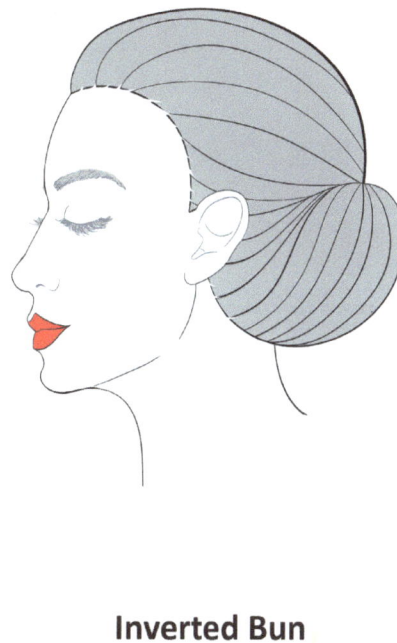

Braided Front Hairline

Side Part

Beachy Waves

Inverted Bun

MEDIUM LENGTH - ROUND BOTTOM

THE ONE LENGTH HAIRCUT

Styling Options with Bangs

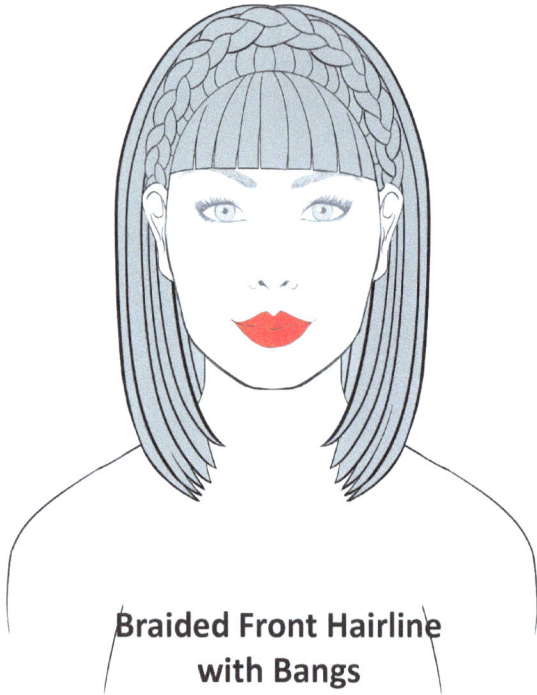

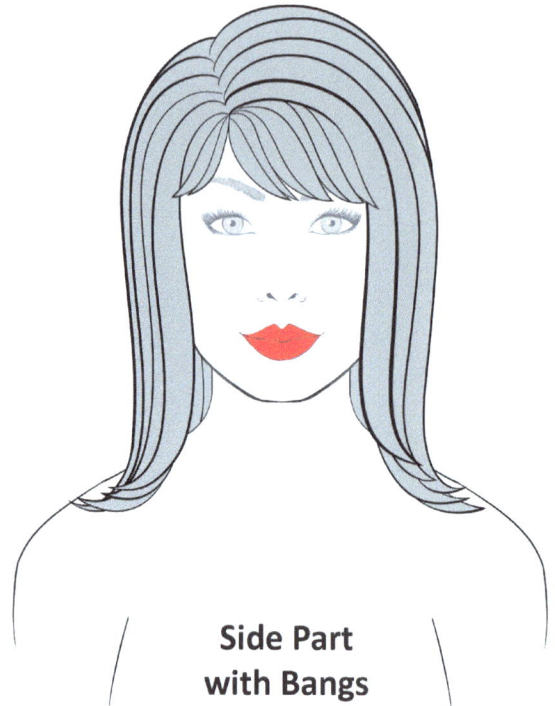

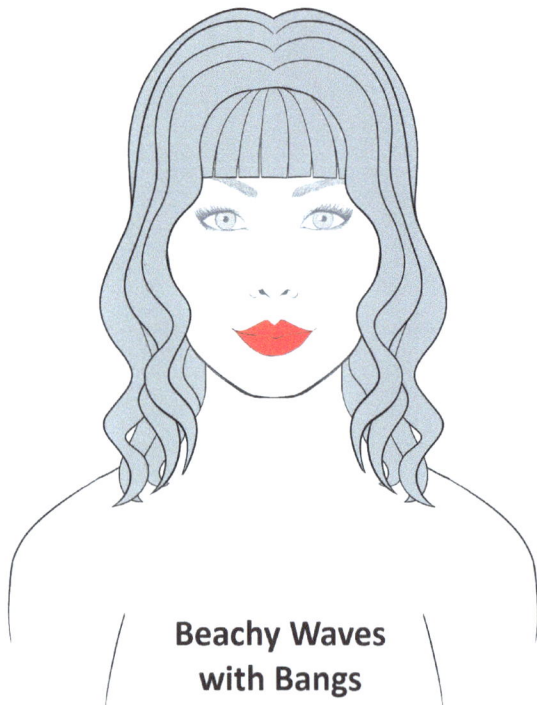

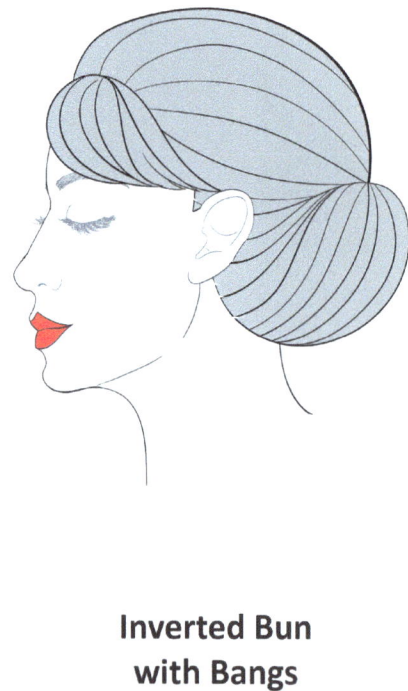

**Braided Front Hairline
with Bangs**

**Side Part
with Bangs**

**Beachy Waves
with Bangs**

**Inverted Bun
with Bangs**

MEDIUM LENGTH - ROUND BOTTOM

THE ONE LENGTH HAIRCUT

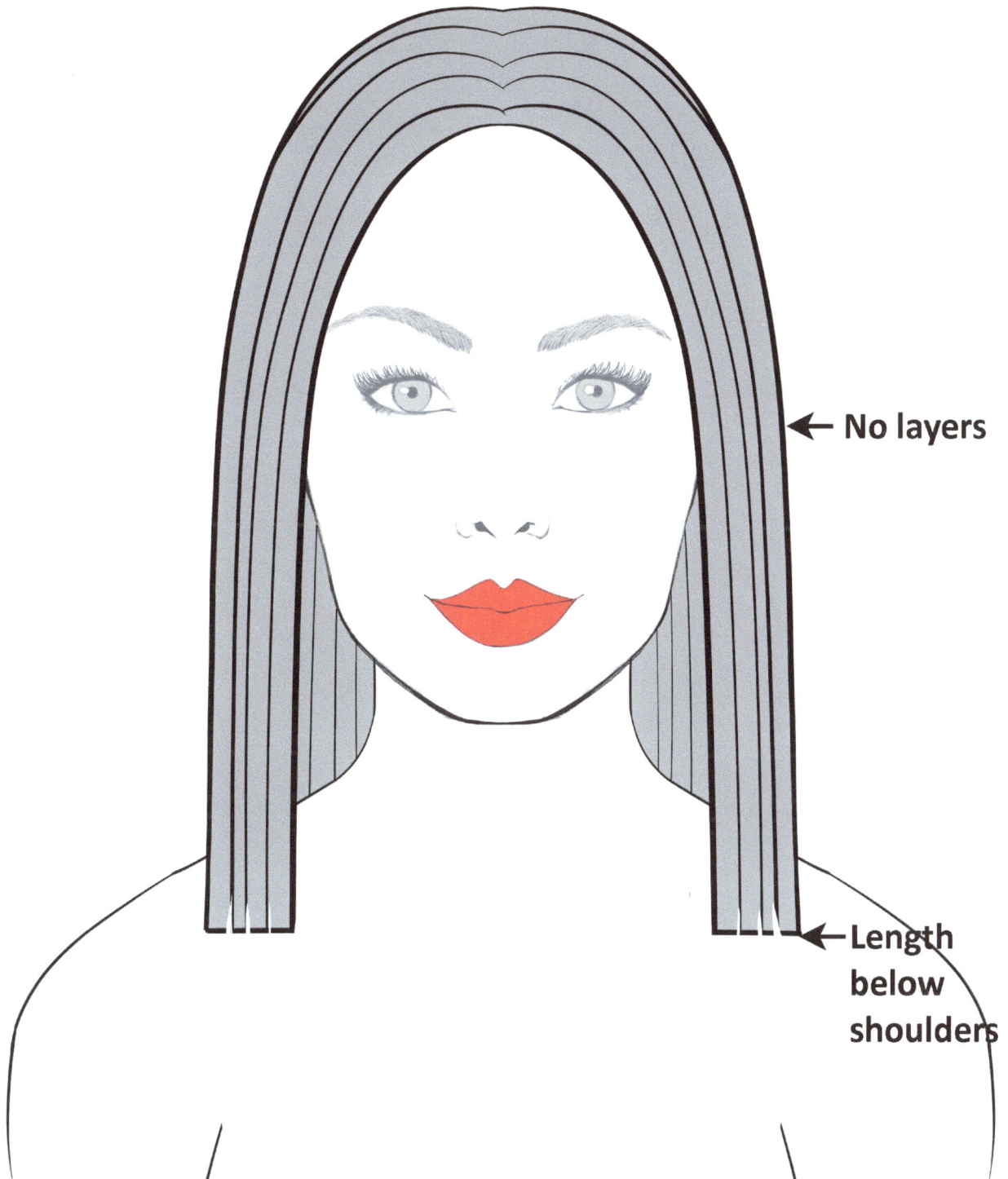

← No layers

← Length below shoulders

MEDIUM LENGTH - STRAIGHT BOTTOM

THE ONE LENGTH HAIRCUT

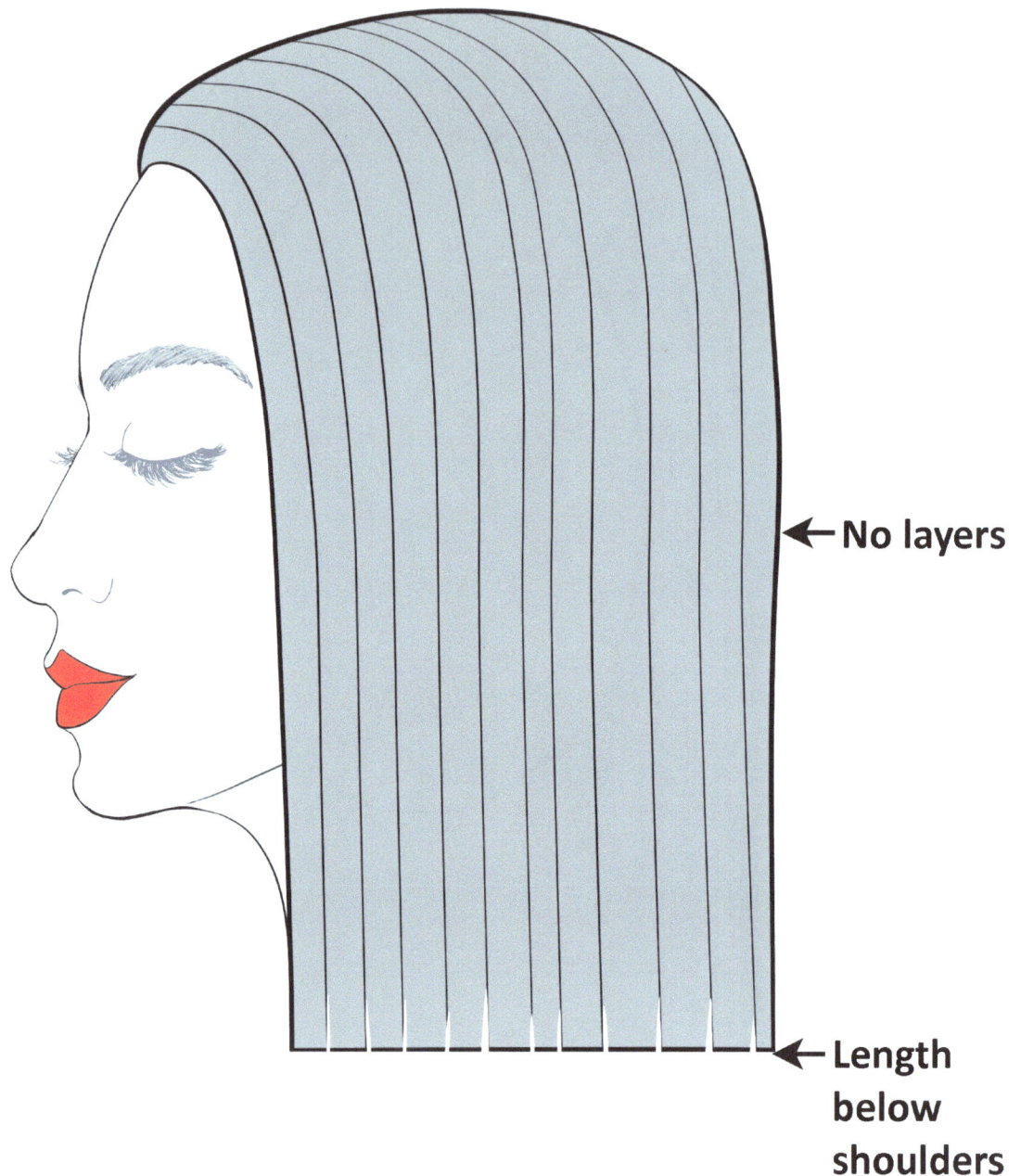

← No layers

← Length below shoulders

MEDIUM LENGTH - STRAIGHT BOTTOM

THE ONE LENGTH HAIRCUT

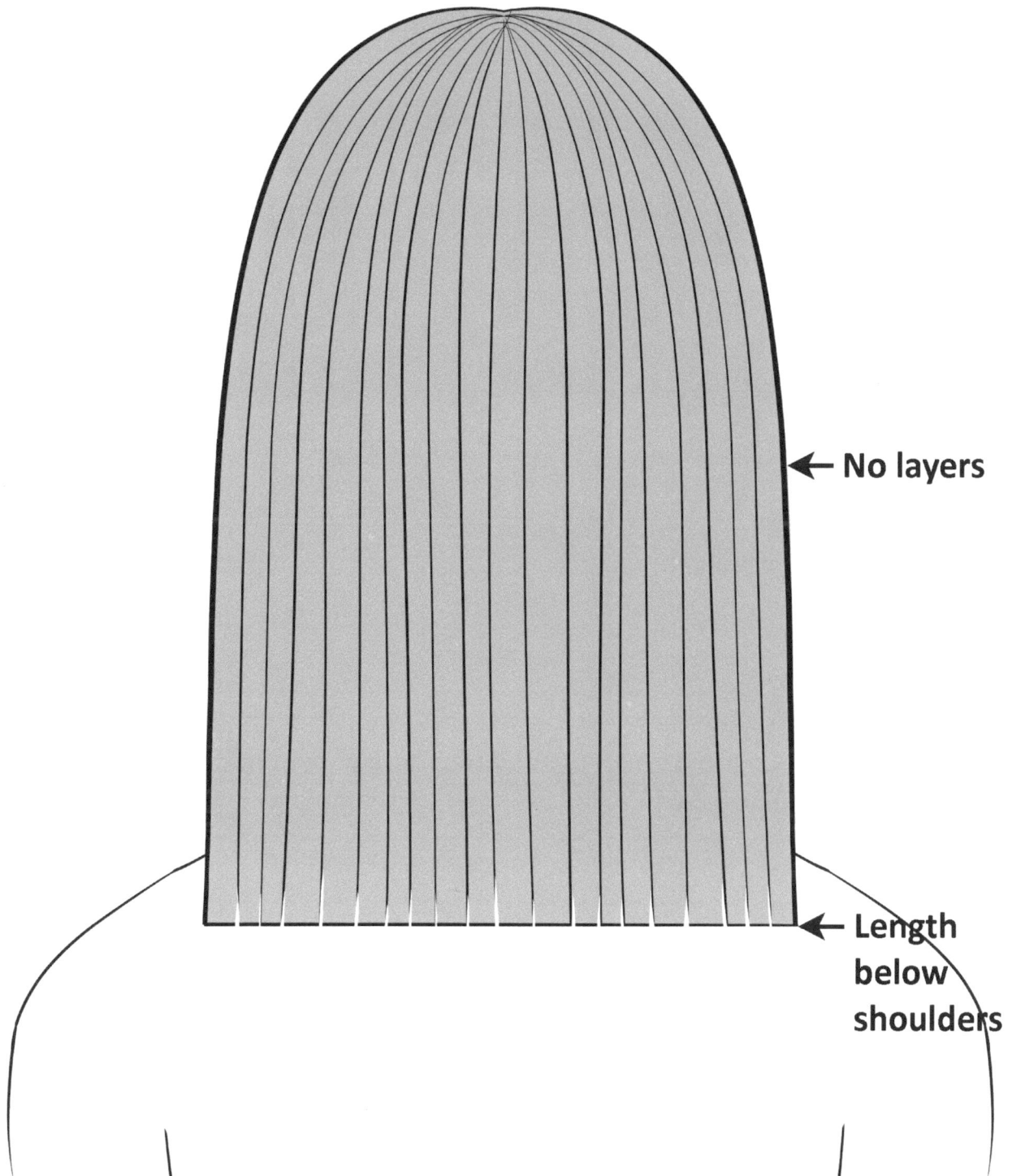

← No layers

← Length
below
shoulders

MEDIUM LENGTH - STRAIGHT BOTTOM

THE ONE LENGTH HAIRCUT

Styling Options

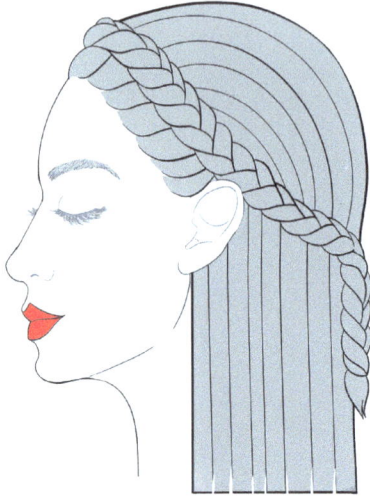

Partially Braided

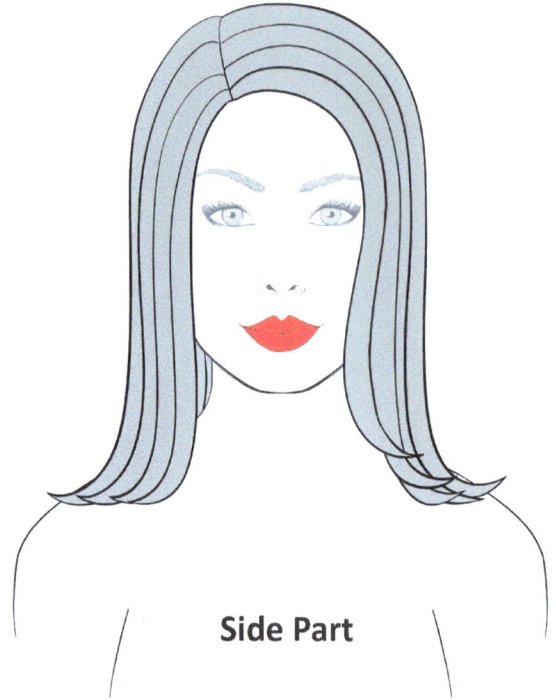

Side Part

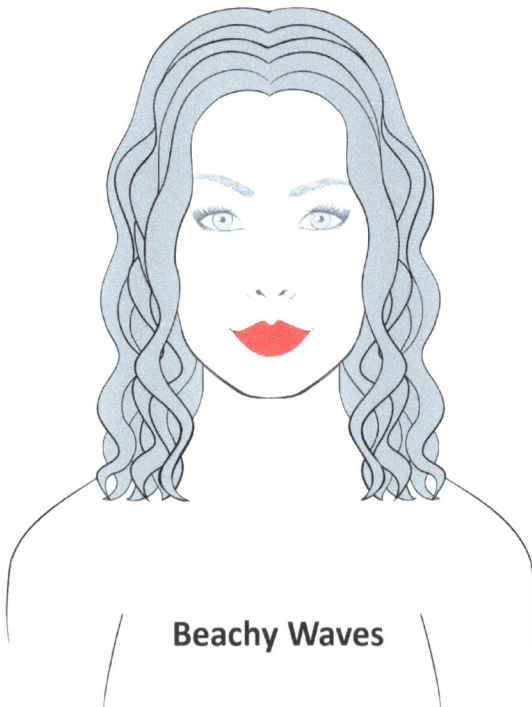

Beachy Waves

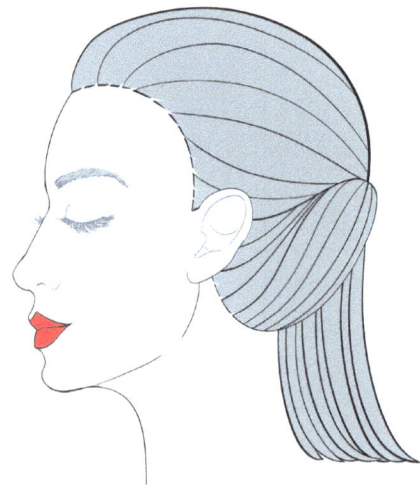

Inverted Ponytail

MEDIUM LENGTH - STRAIGHT BOTTOM

THE ONE LENGTH HAIRCUT

Styling Options with Bangs

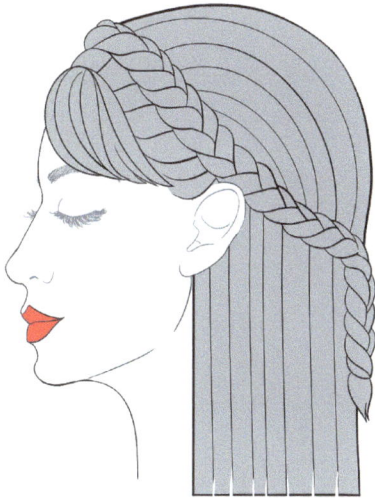

**Partially Braided
with Bangs**

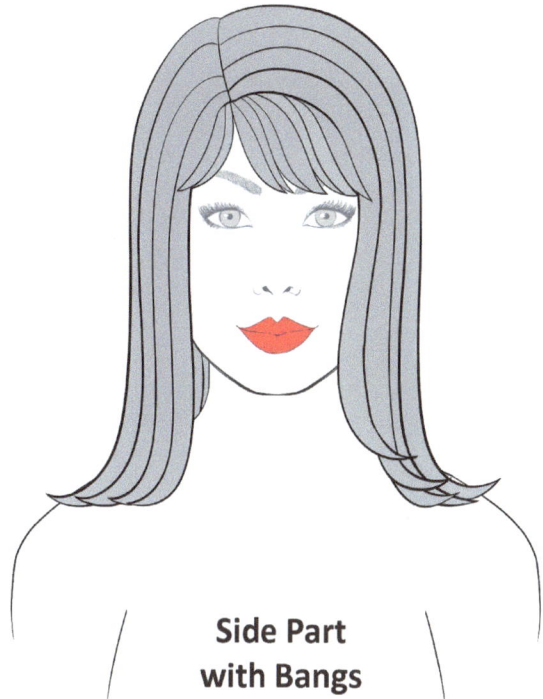

**Side Part
with Bangs**

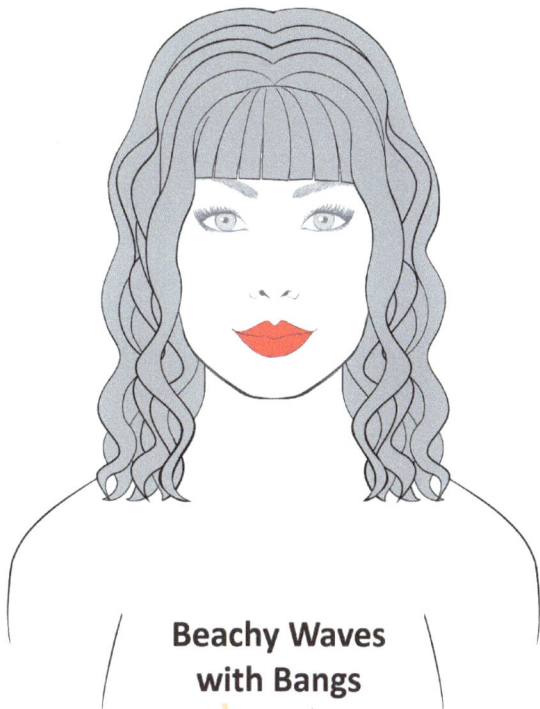

**Beachy Waves
with Bangs**

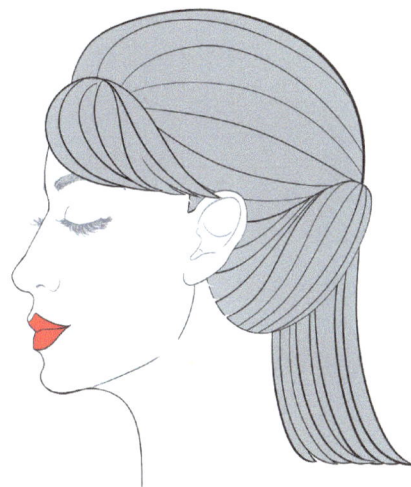

**Inverted Ponytail
with Bangs**

MEDIUM LENGTH - STRAIGHT BOTTOM

THE ONE LENGTH HAIRCUT

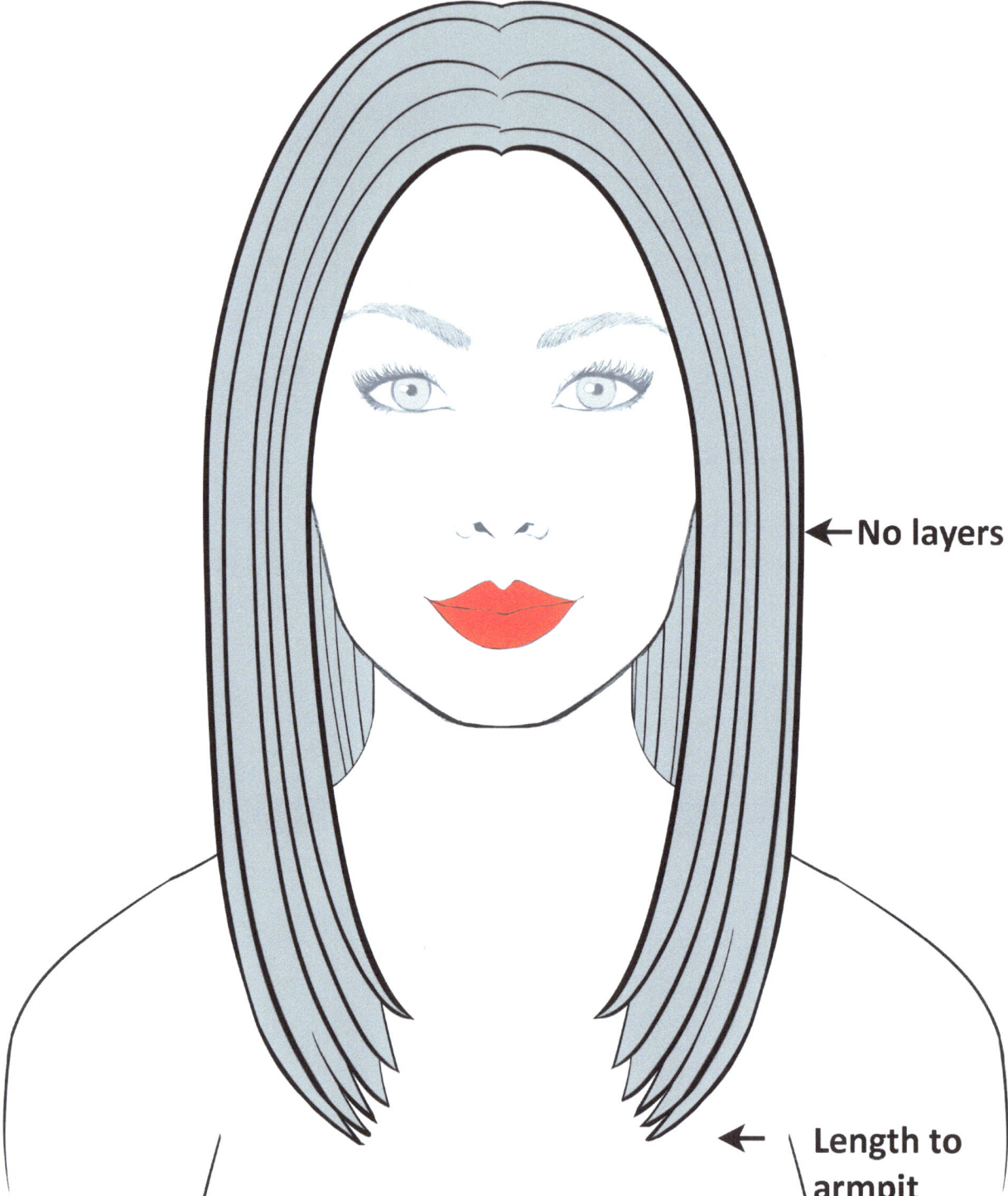

← No layers

← Length to armpit

LONG LENGTH - ROUND BOTTOM

THE ONE LENGTH HAIRCUT

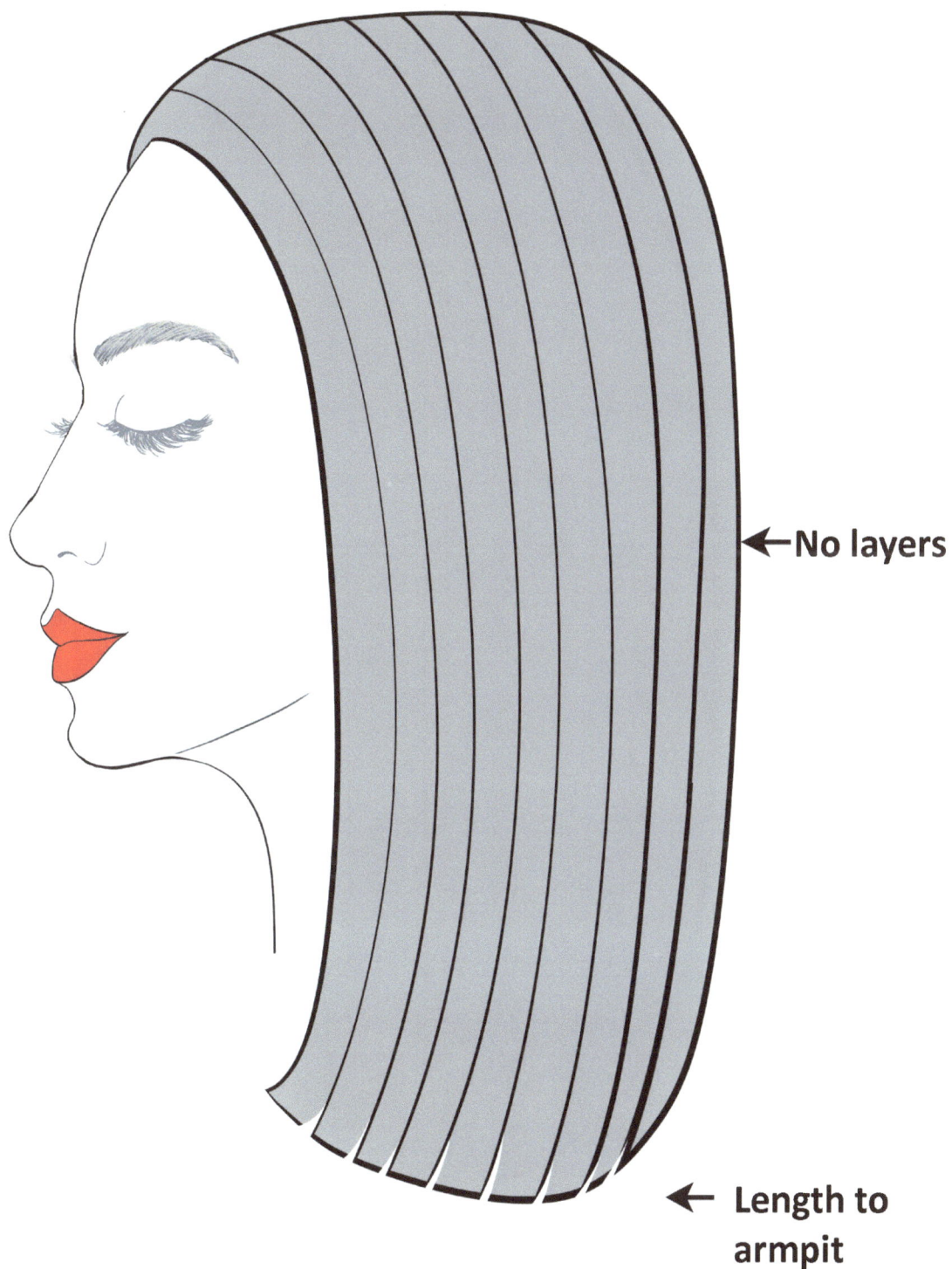

← No layers

← Length to armpit

LONG LENGTH - ROUND BOTTOM

THE ONE LENGTH HAIRCUT

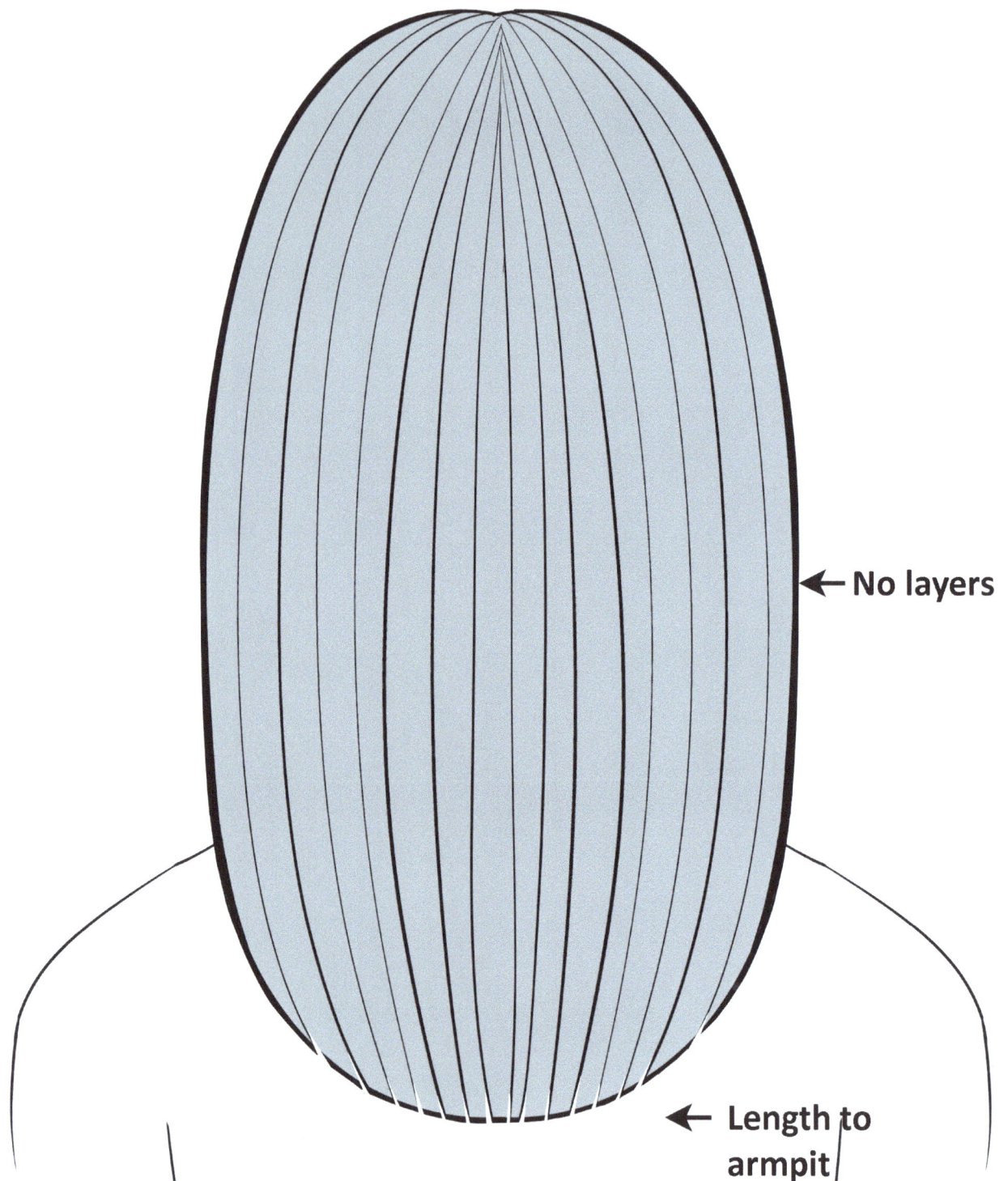

← No layers

← Length to armpit

LONG LENGTH - ROUND BOTTOM

THE ONE LENGTH HAIRCUT

Styling Options

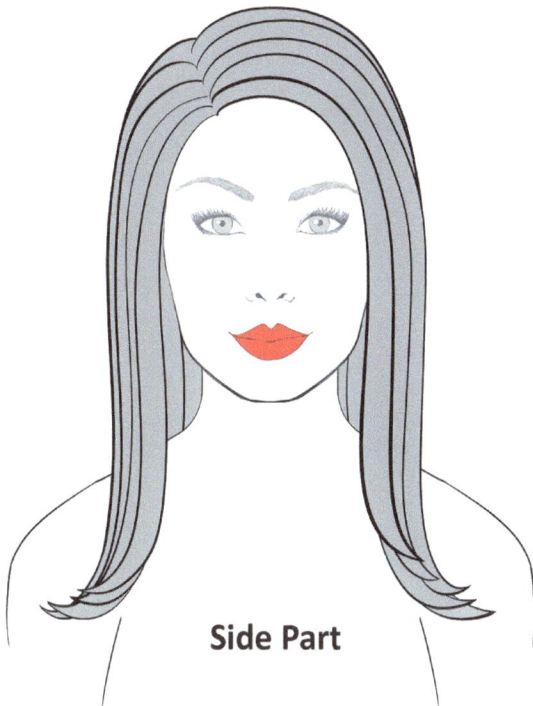

Side Part

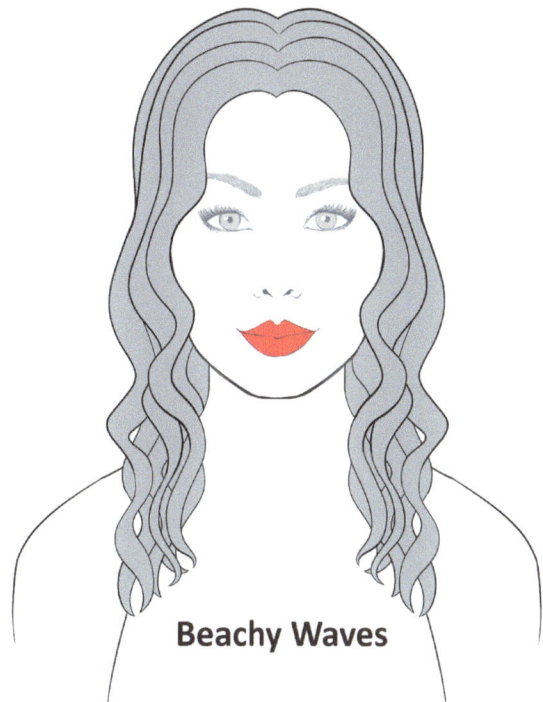

Beachy Waves

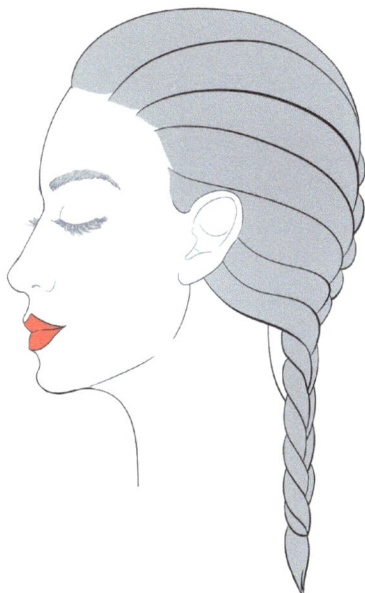

French Braid

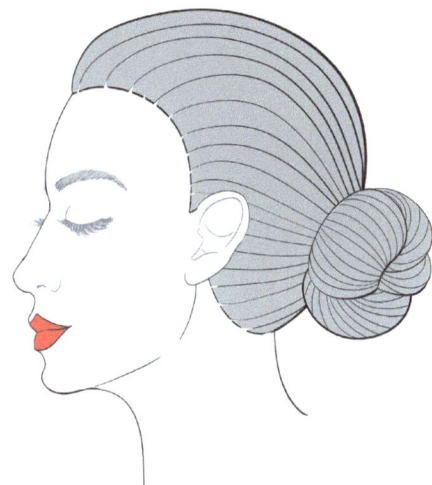

Bun

LONG LENGTH - ROUND BOTTOM

THE ONE LENGTH HAIRCUT

Styling Options with Bangs

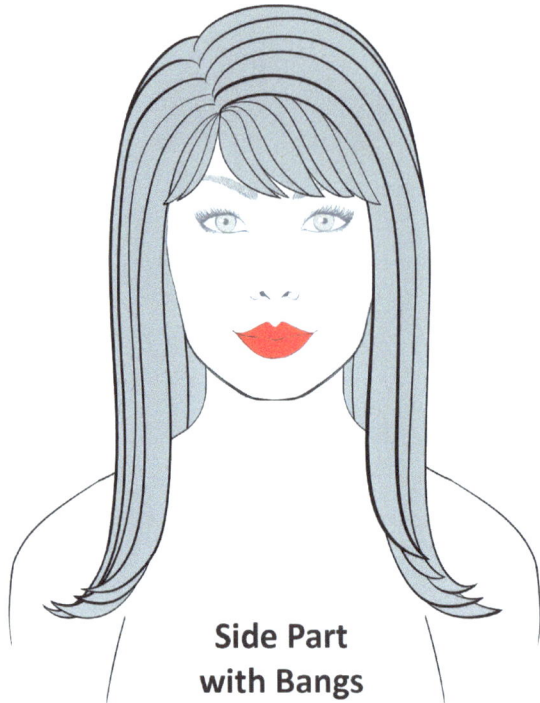

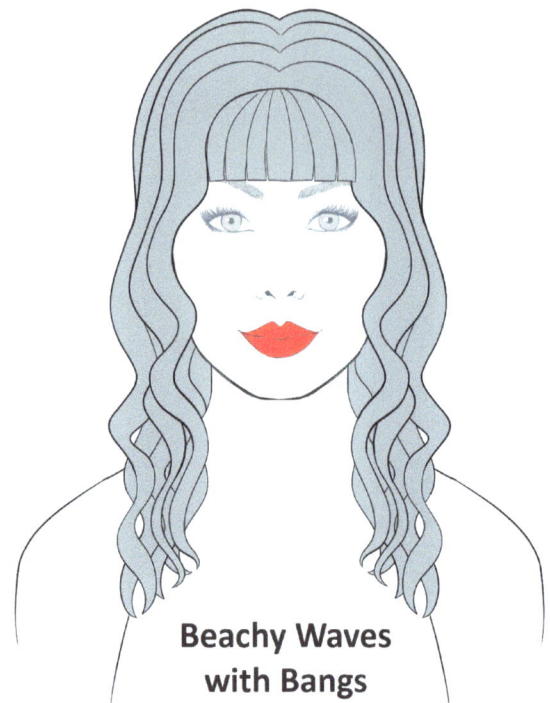

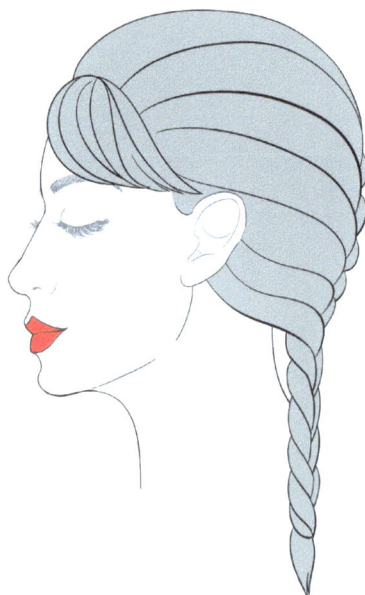

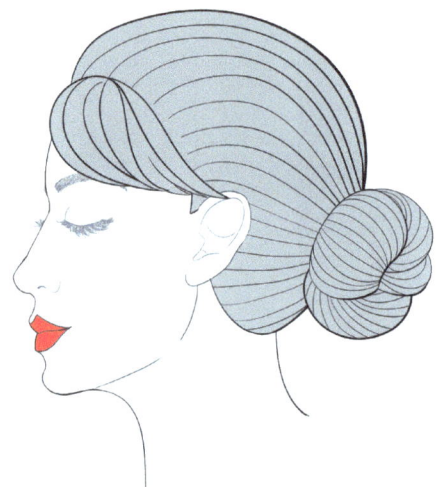

**Side Part
with Bangs**

**Beachy Waves
with Bangs**

**French Braid
with Bangs**

**Bun
with Bangs**

LONG LENGTH - ROUND BOTTOM

THE ONE LENGTH HAIRCUT

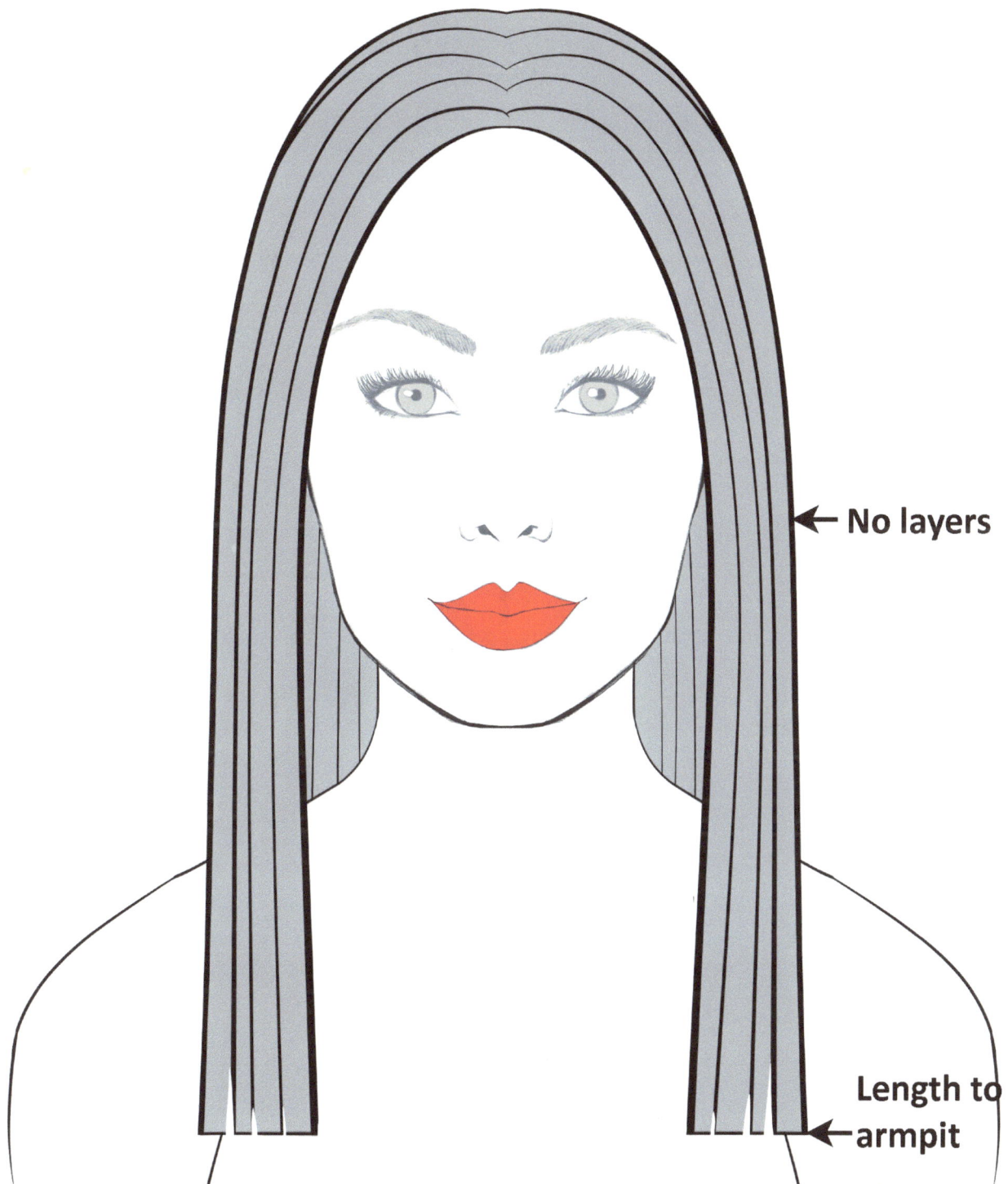

← No layers

Length to ← armpit

LONG LENGTH - STRAIGHT BOTTOM

THE ONE LENGTH HAIRCUT

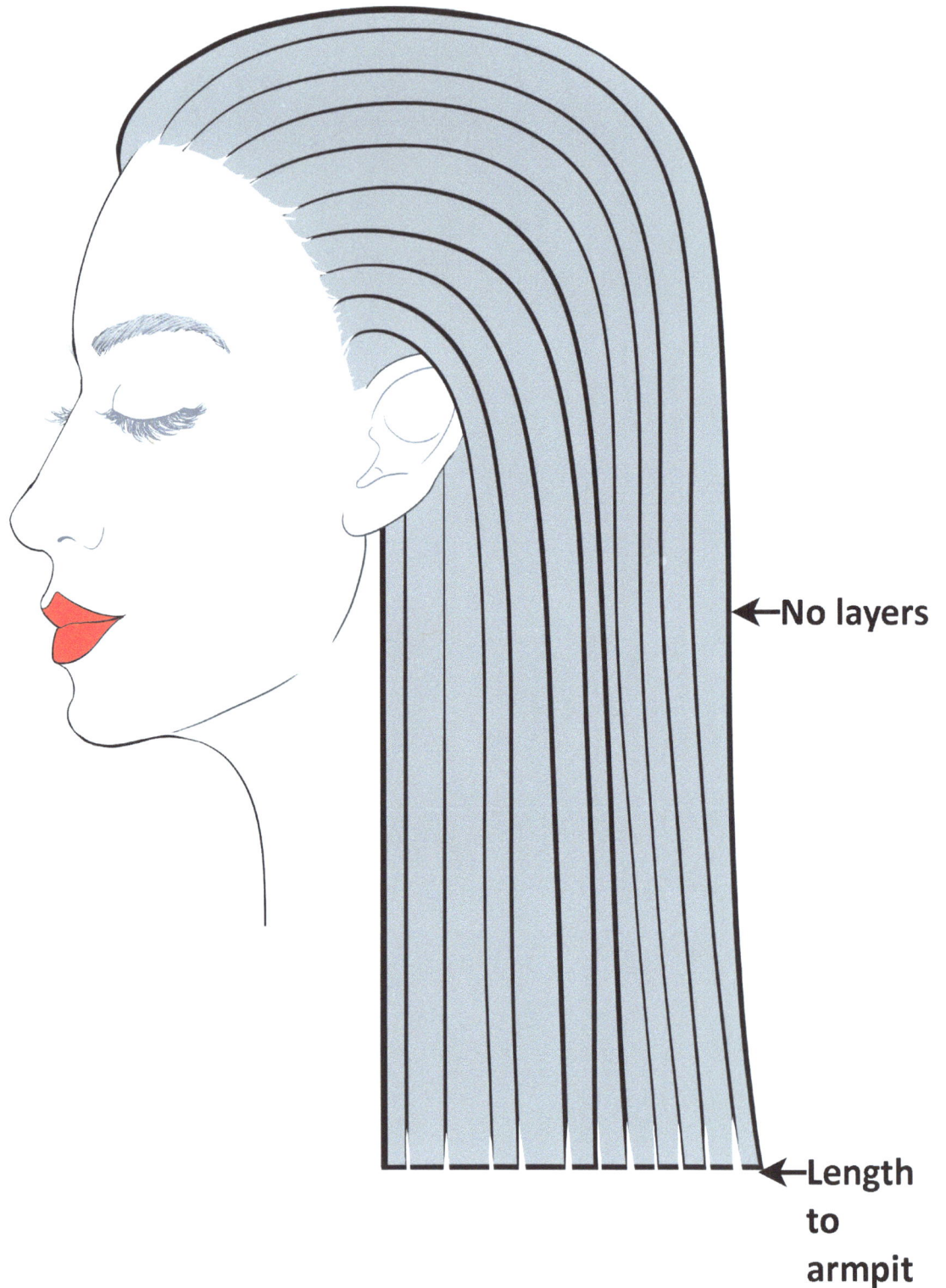

← No layers

← Length to armpit

LONG LENGTH - STRAIGHT BOTTOM

THE ONE LENGTH HAIRCUT

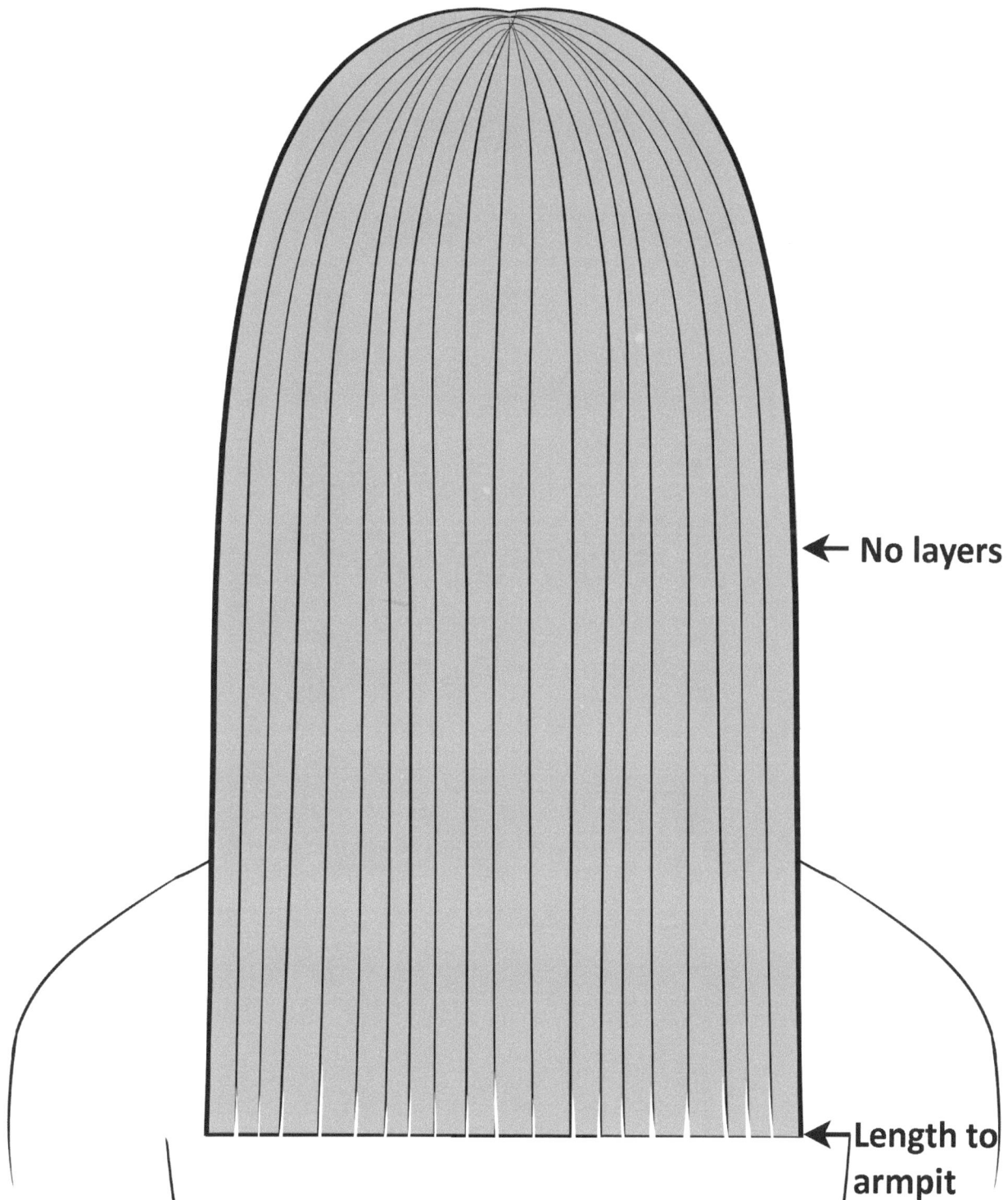

← No layers

← Length to armpit

LONG LENGTH - STRAIGHT BOTTOM

THE ONE LENGTH HAIRCUT

Styling Options

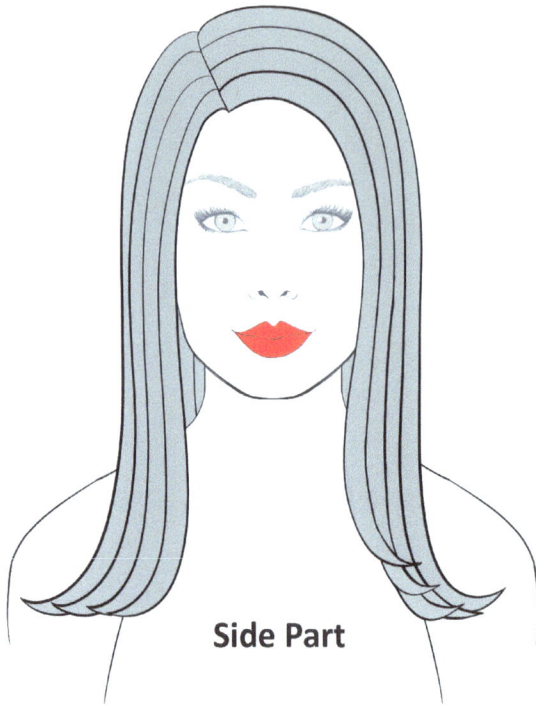

Side Part

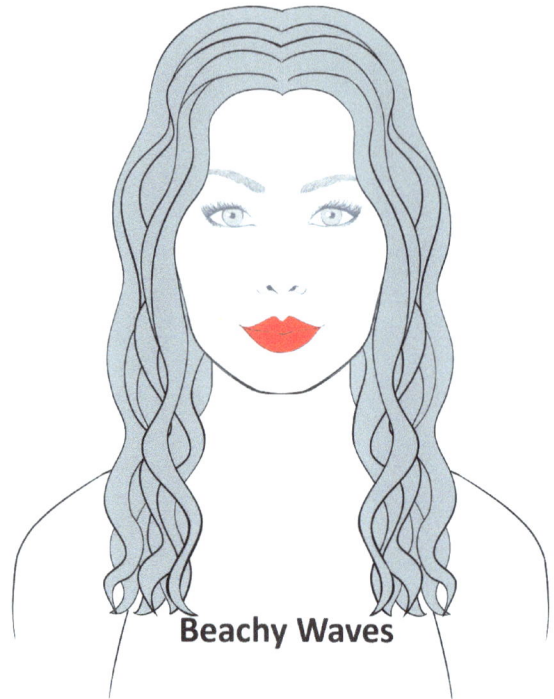

Beachy Waves

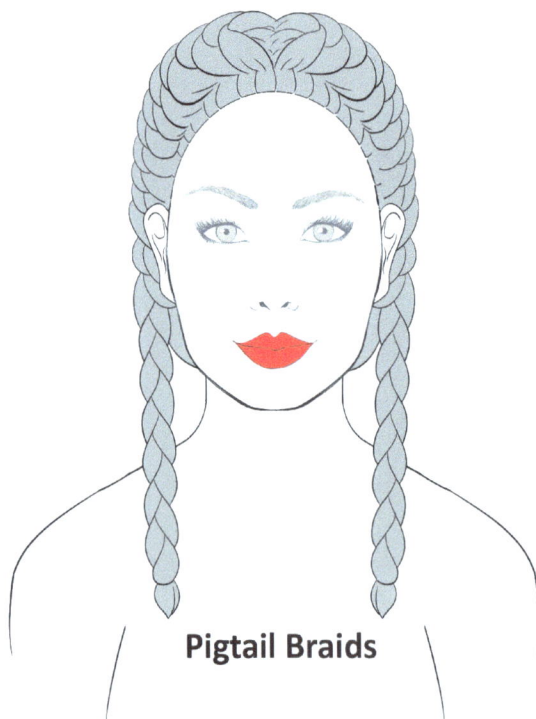

Pigtail Braids

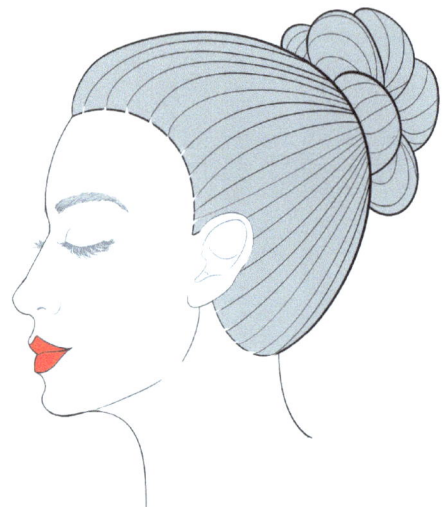

Up-Do

LONG LENGTH - STRAIGHT BOTTOM

THE ONE LENGTH HAIRCUT

Styling Options with Bangs

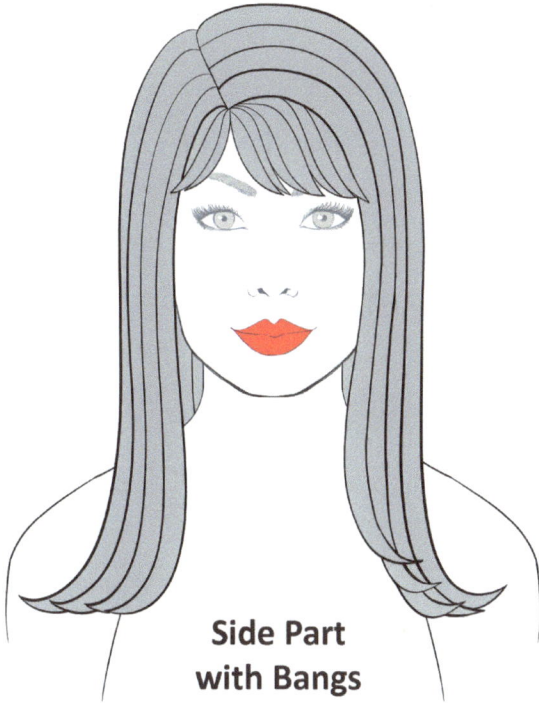

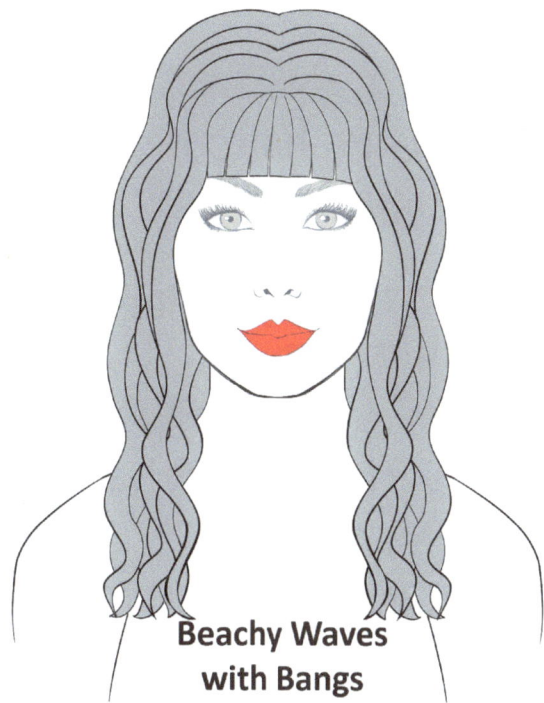

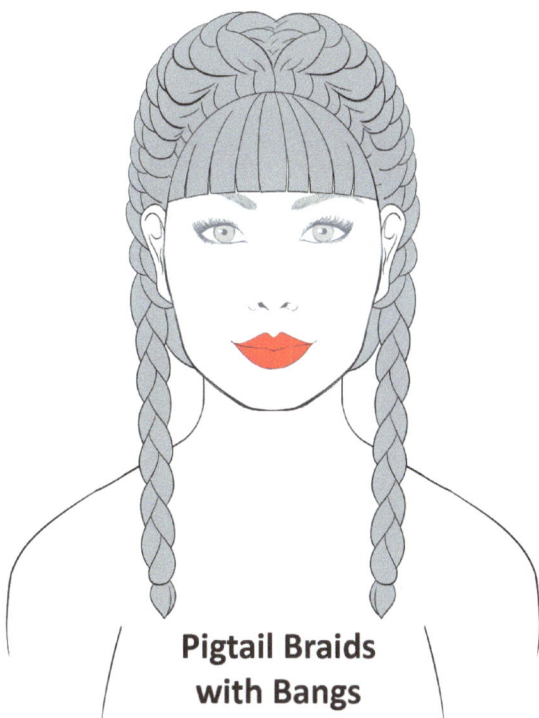

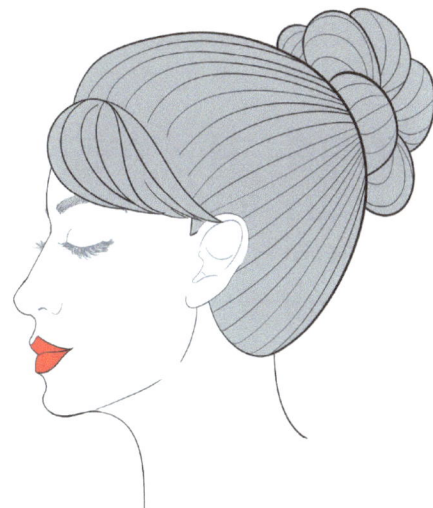

**Side Part
with Bangs**

**Beachy Waves
with Bangs**

**Pigtail Braids
with Bangs**

**Up-Do
with Bangs**

LONG LENGTH - STRAIGHT BOTTOM

Chapter 3
THE A-LINE HAIRCUT

This super fun haircut offers the illusion of length and has a modern vibe.

- **LENGTH-** The A-Line Haircut looks great in short lengths and medium lengths.

- **PART-** This haircut has a fixed part and is not interchangeable.

- **BANGS-** Looks great with or without bangs.

- **LAYERS-** Choose light layers or no layers to serve your unique hair texture and hair type.

- **STYLING-** The A-Line Haircut is effortless to style. Simply blow dry and if needed use a flat iron for a polished finish. For those with wavy or curly hair type apply product and let your hair dry naturally.

THE A-LINE HAIRCUT

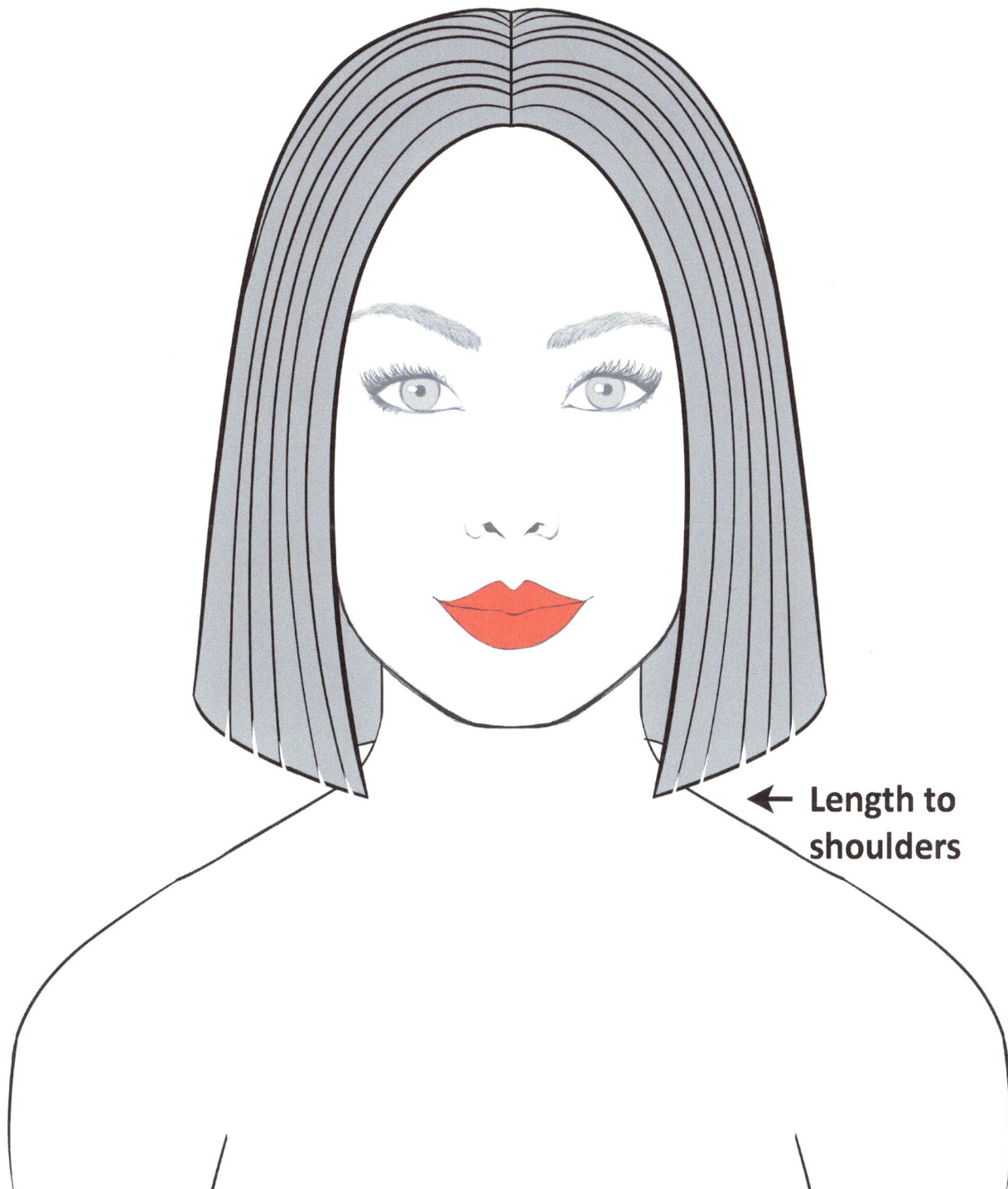

← **Length to shoulders**

SHORT LENGTH - CENTER PART

THE A-LINE HAIRCUT

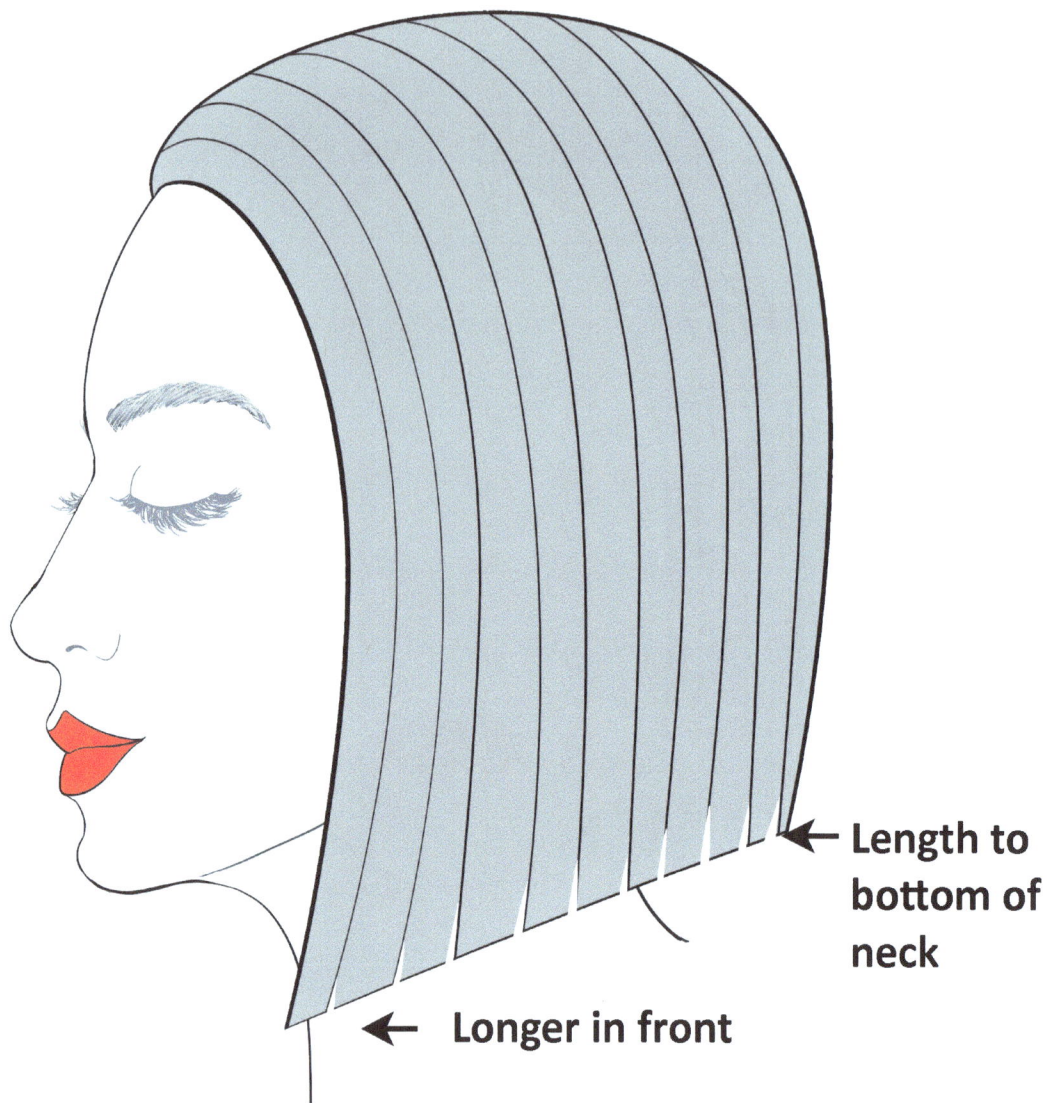

← Length to bottom of neck

← Longer in front

SHORT LENGTH - CENTER PART

THE A-LINE HAIRCUT

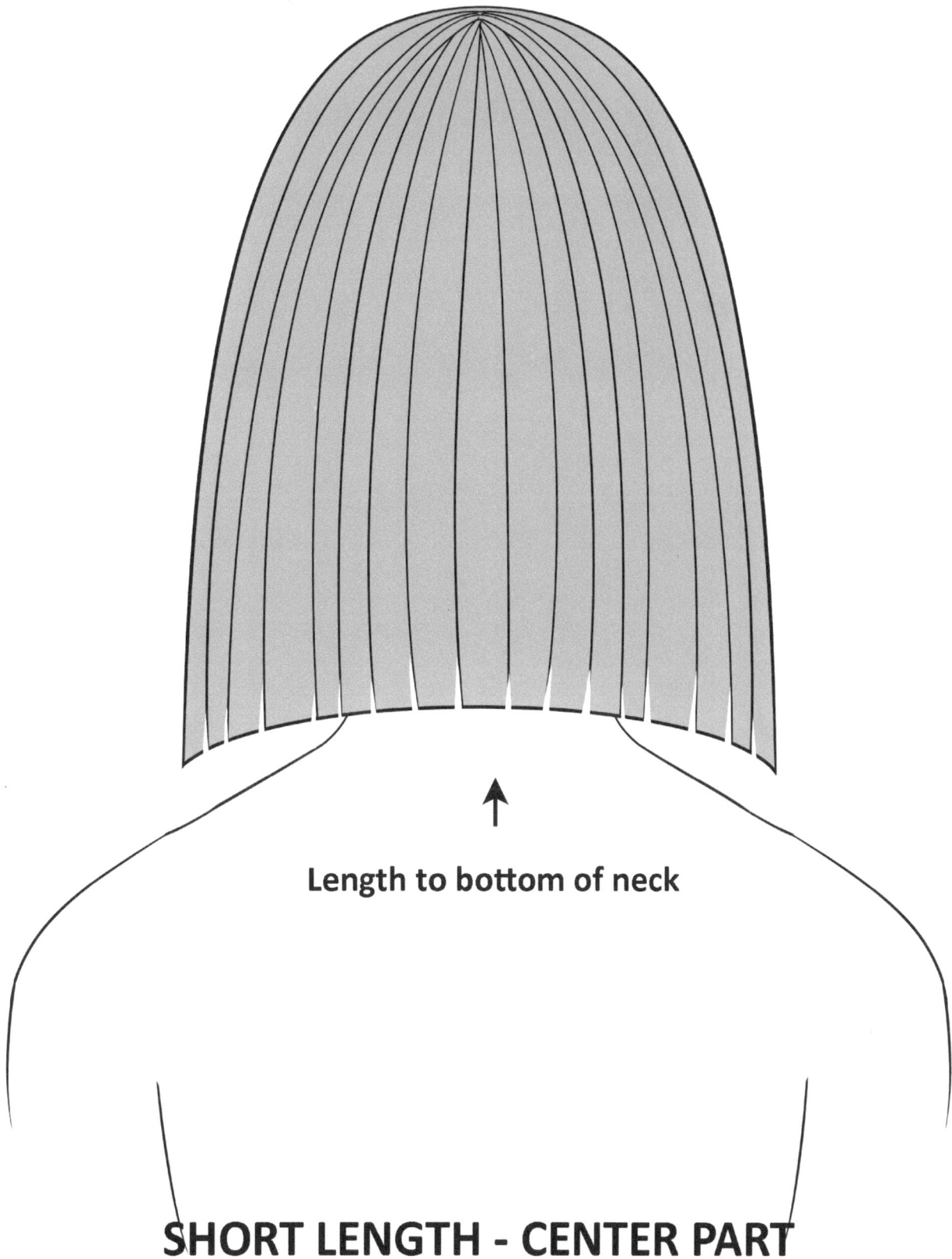

Length to bottom of neck

SHORT LENGTH - CENTER PART

THE A-LINE HAIRCUT

Disconnected Bang Options

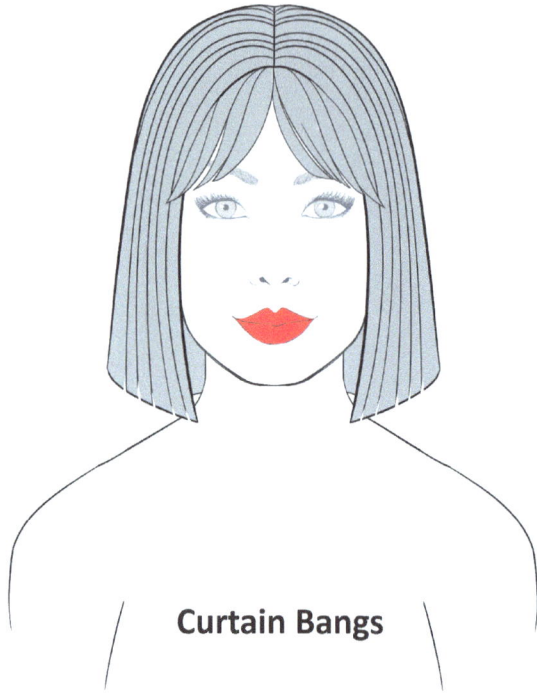

Curtain Bangs

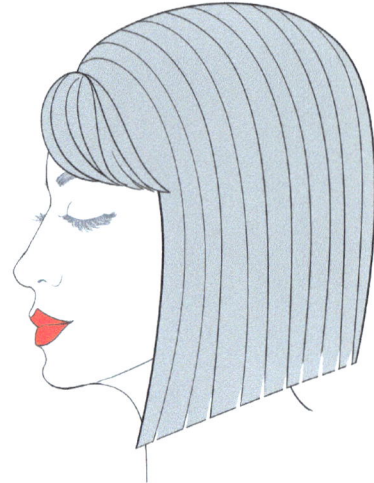

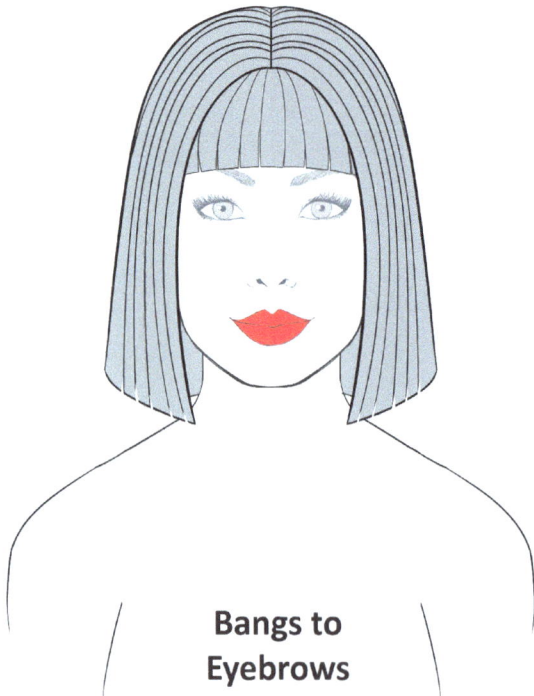

Curtain Bangs

Bangs to Eyebrows

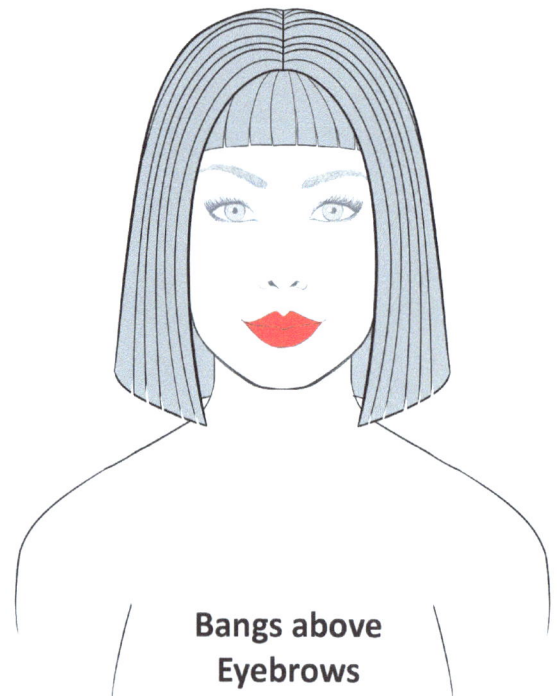

Bangs above Eyebrows

SHORT LENGTH - CENTER PART

THE A-LINE HAIRCUT

Curly Version

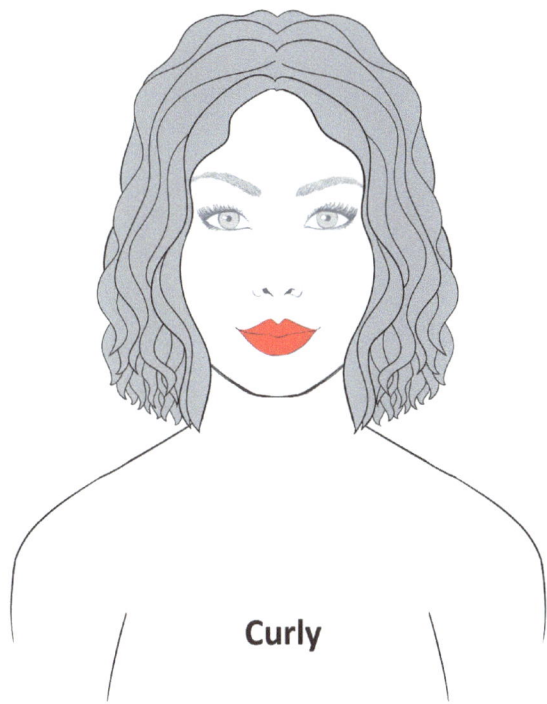

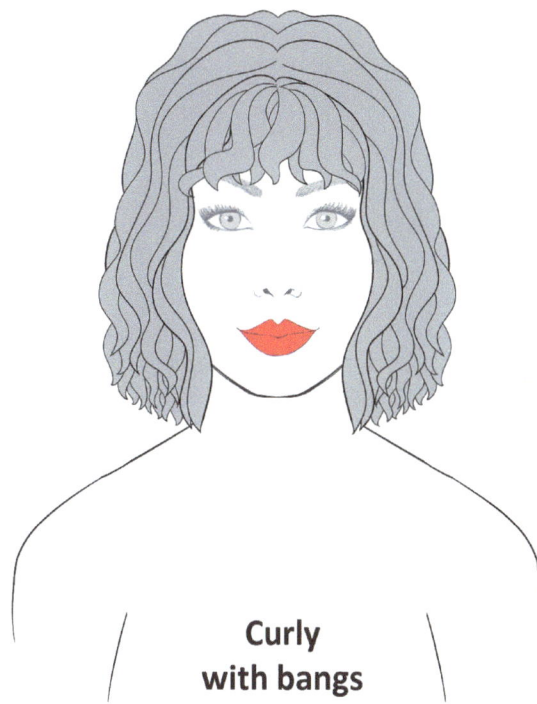

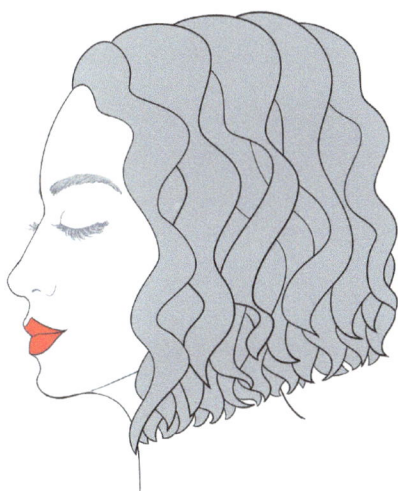

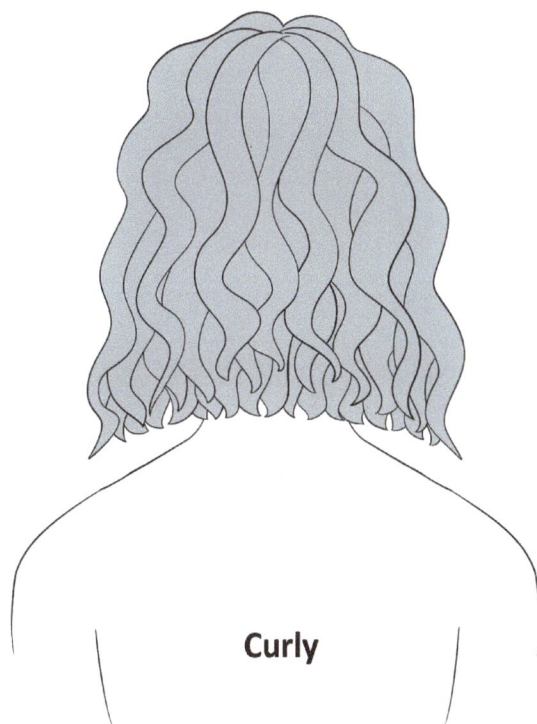

Curly

Curly
with bangs

Curly

Curly

SHORT LENGTH - CENTER PART

THE A-LINE HAIRCUT

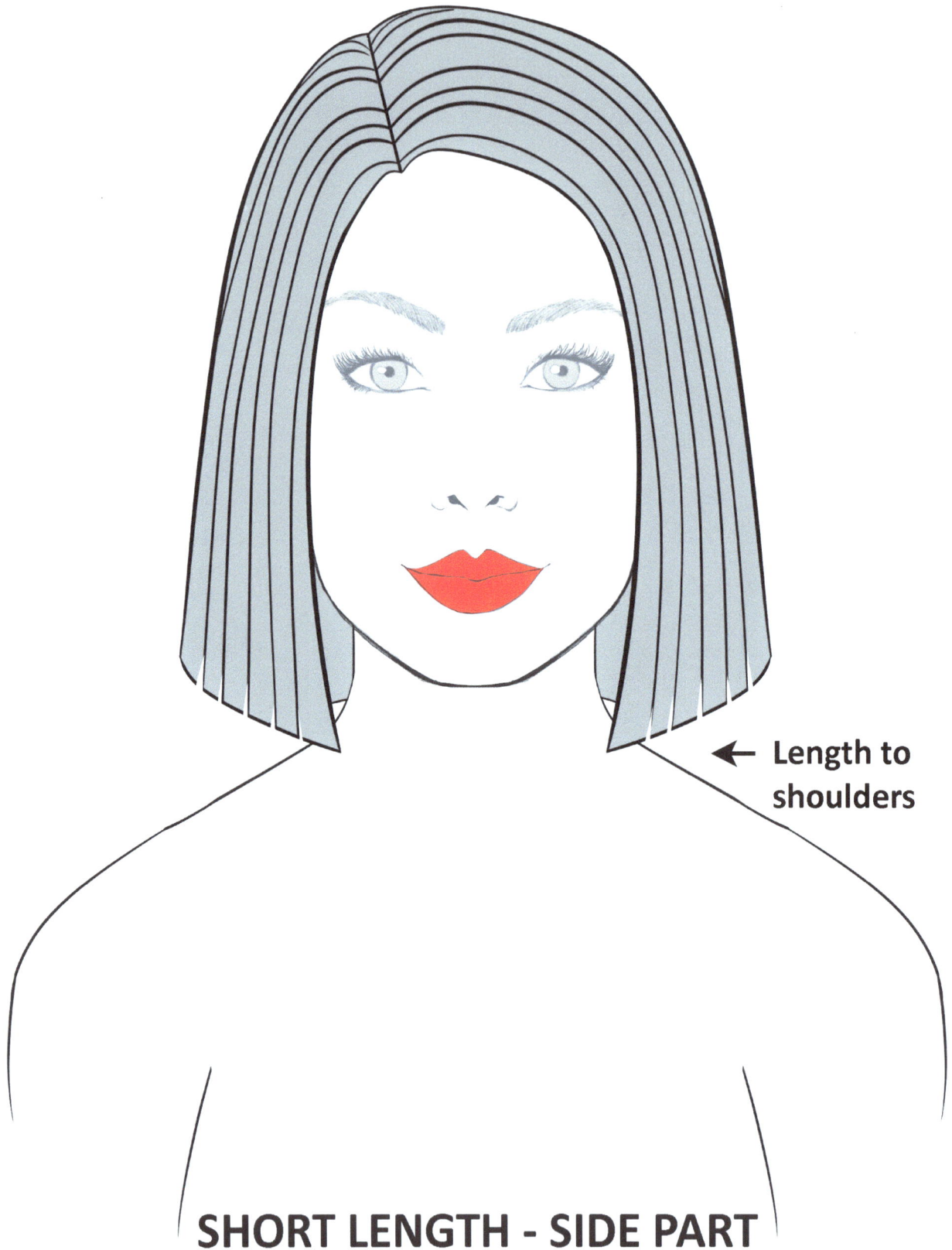

← **Length to shoulders**

SHORT LENGTH - SIDE PART

THE A-LINE HAIRCUT

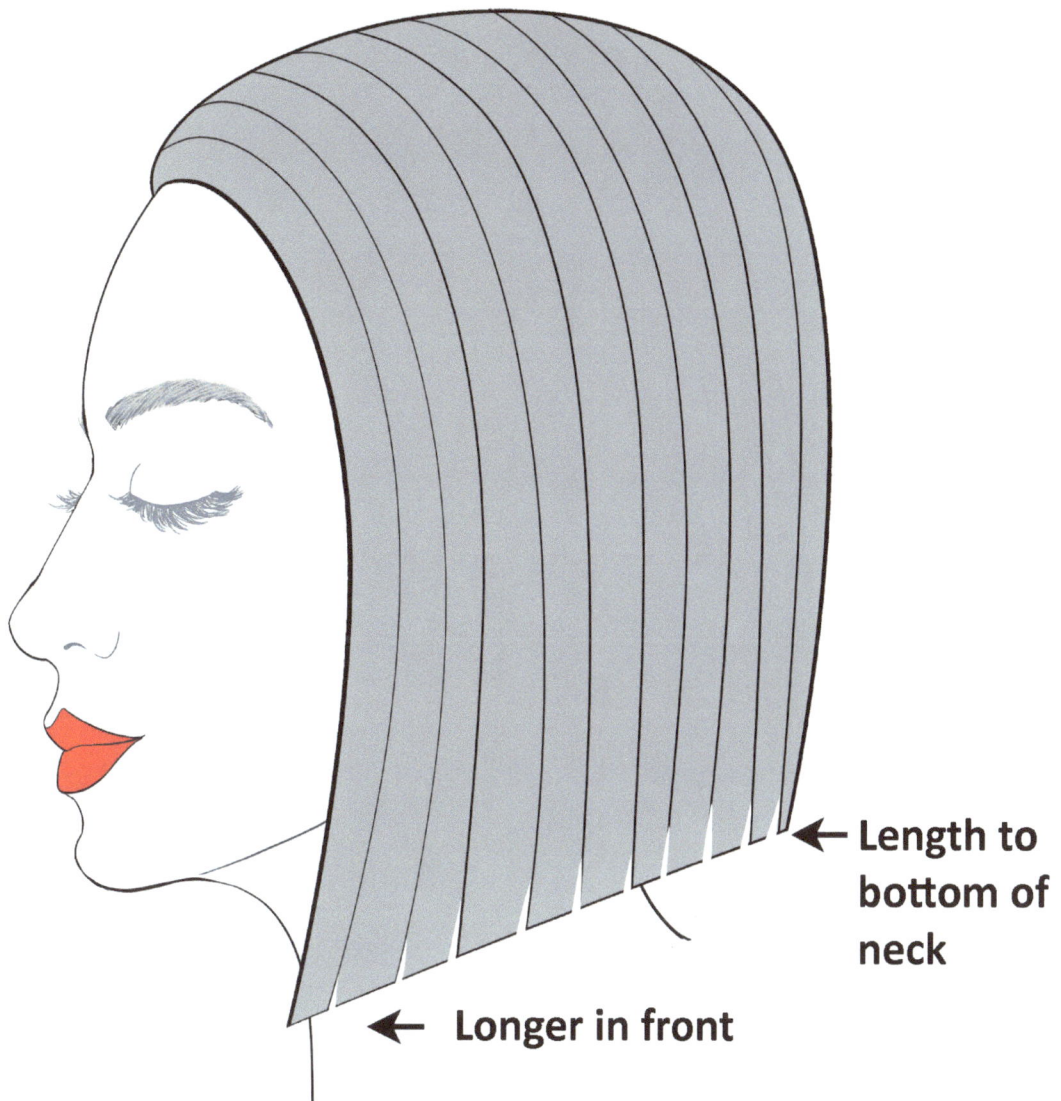

← **Length to bottom of neck**

← **Longer in front**

SHORT LENGTH - SIDE PART

THE A-LINE HAIRCUT

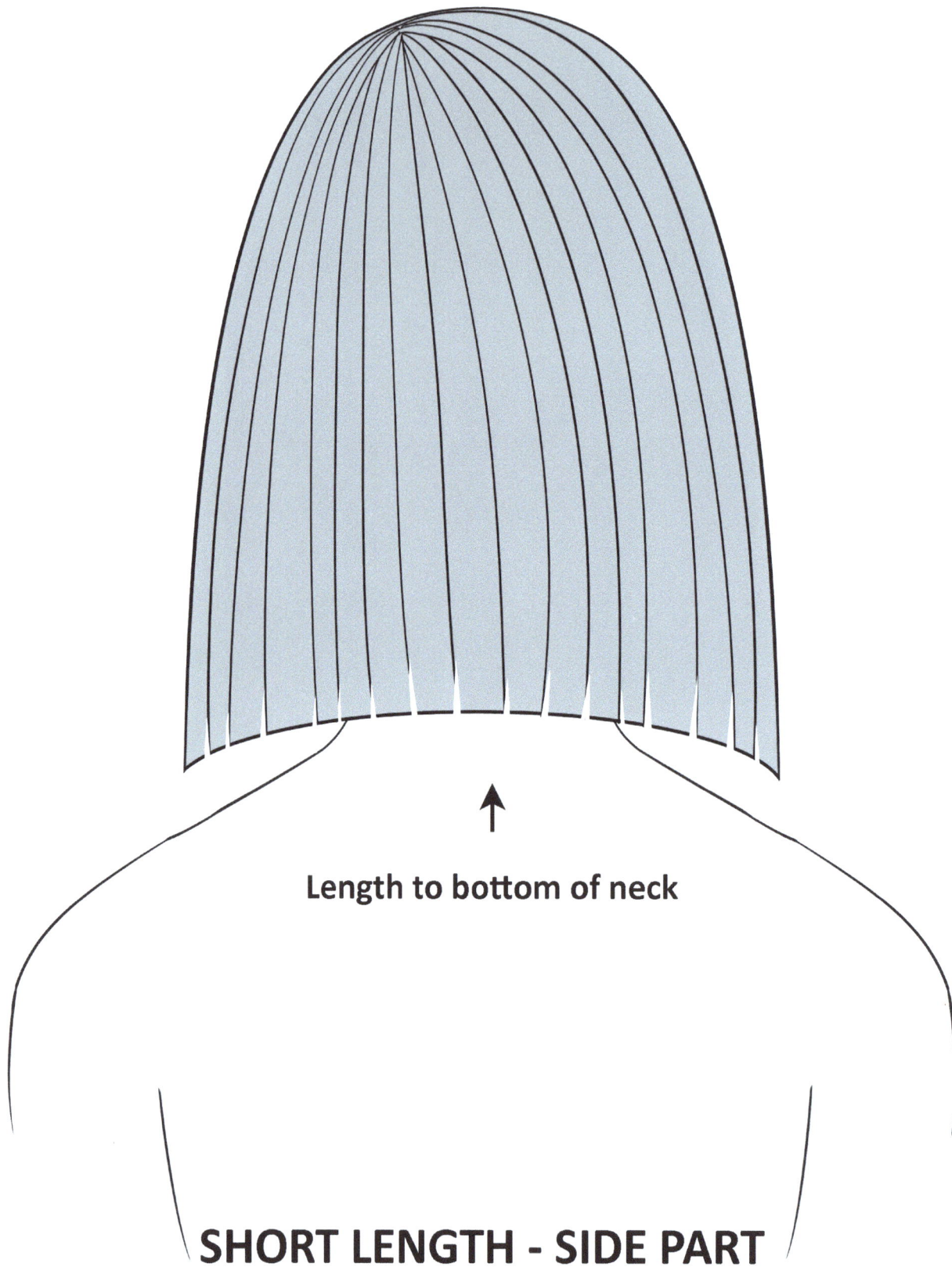

Length to bottom of neck

SHORT LENGTH - SIDE PART

THE A-LINE HAIRCUT

Disconnected Bang Options

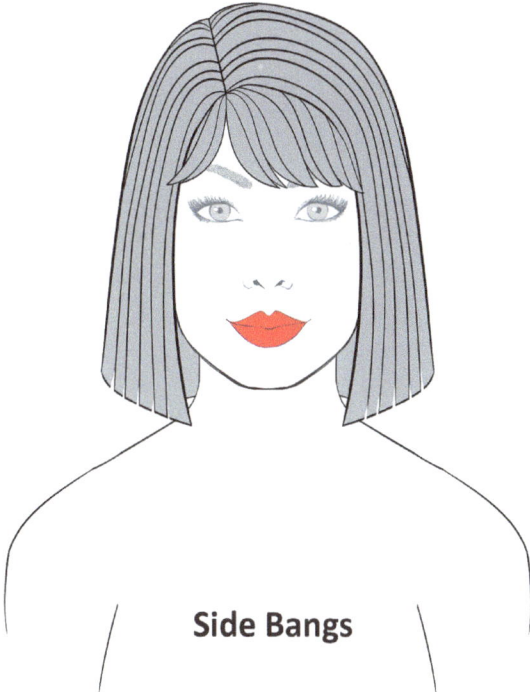

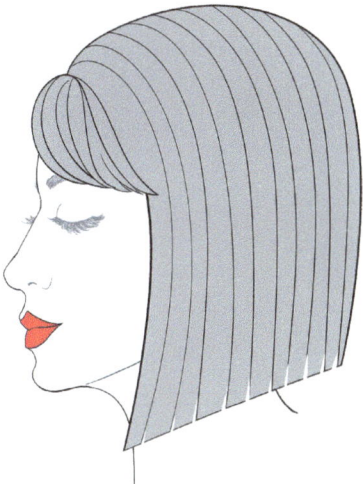

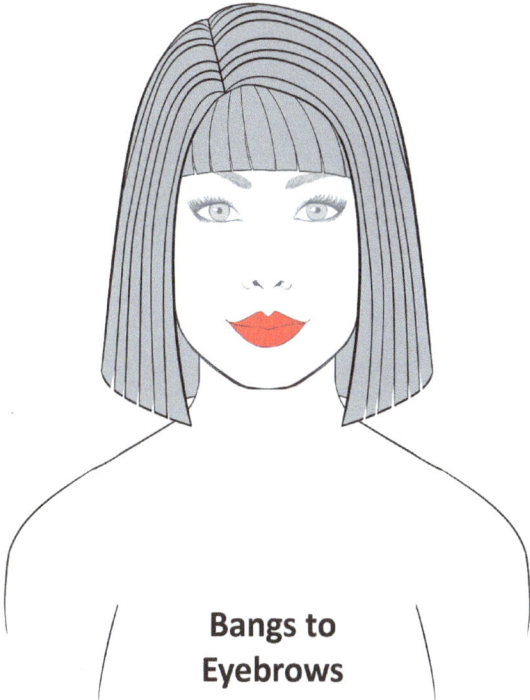

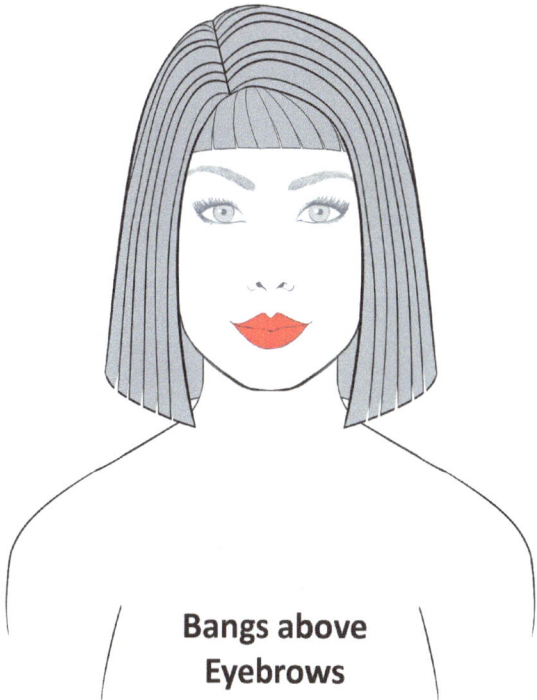

Side Bangs

Side Bangs

Bangs to
Eyebrows

Bangs above
Eyebrows

SHORT LENGTH - SIDE PART

THE A-LINE HAIRCUT

Curly Version

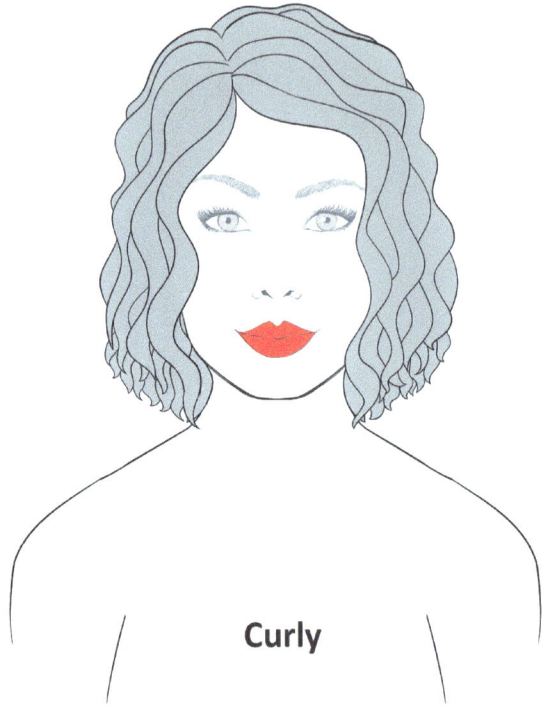

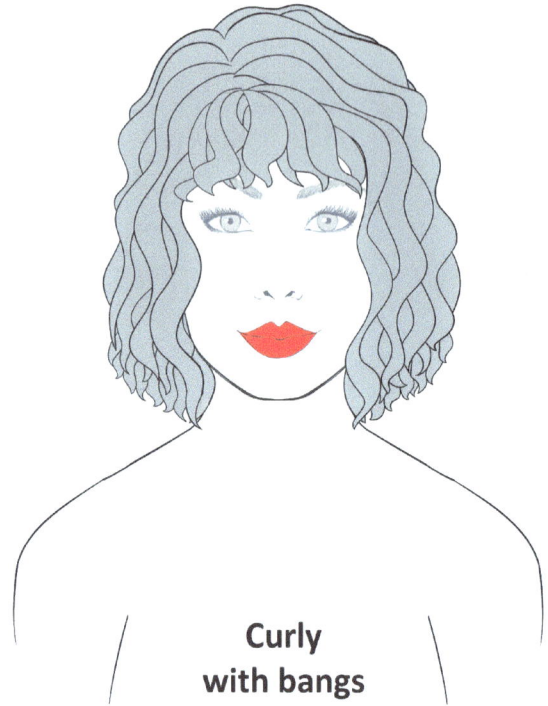

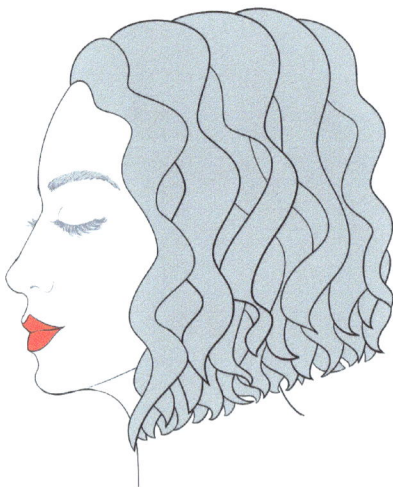

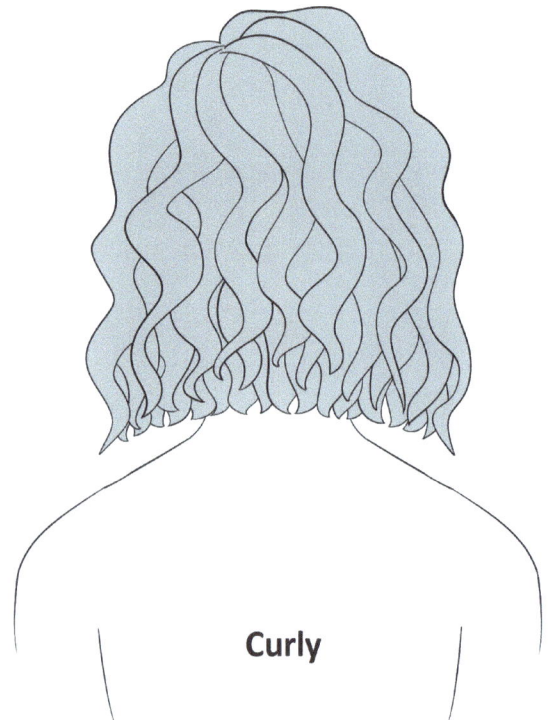

Curly

Curly
with bangs

Curly

Curly

SHORT LENGTH - SIDE PART

THE A-LINE HAIRCUT

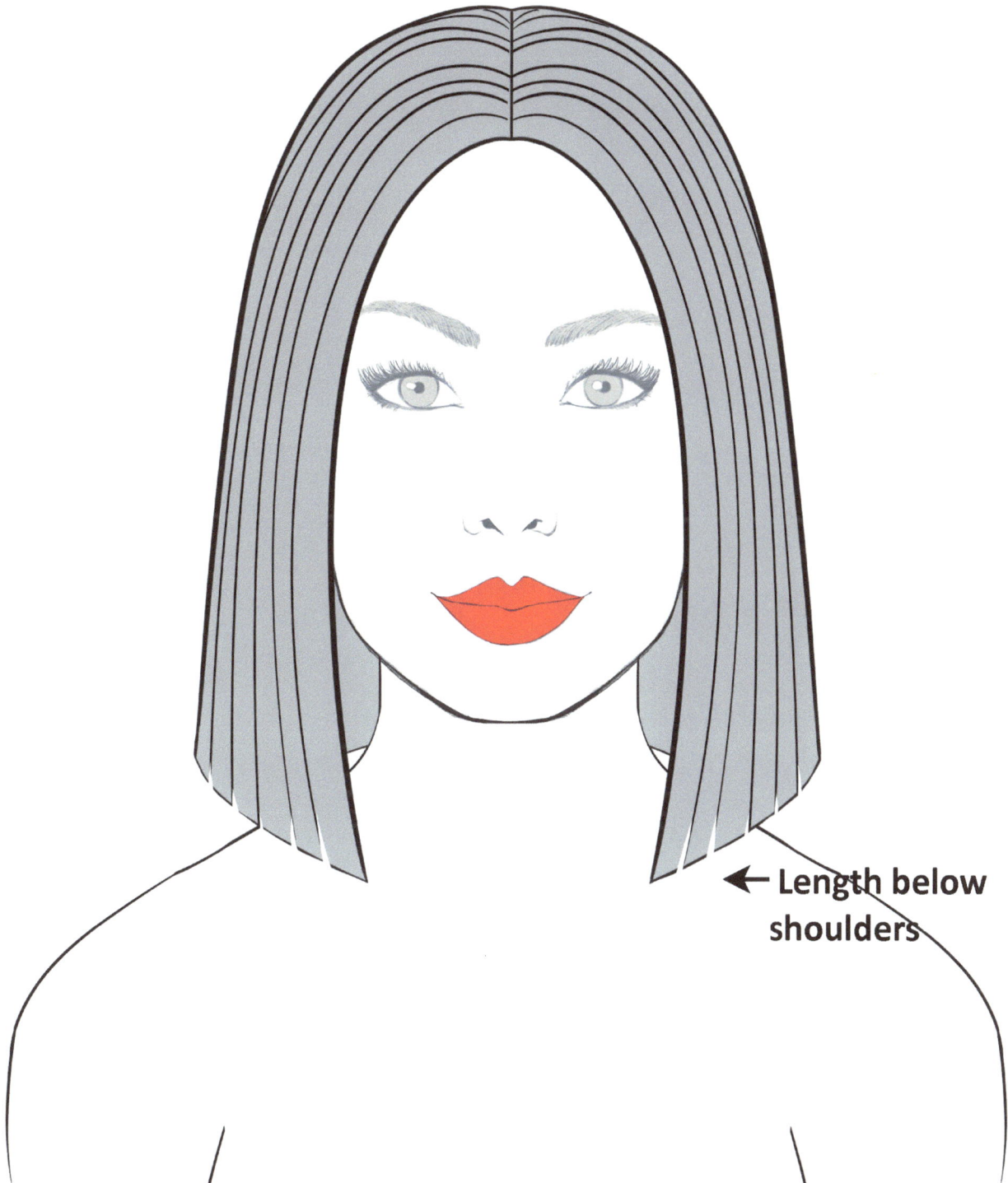

← Length below
shoulders

MEDIUM LENGTH - CENTER PART

THE A-LINE HAIRCUT

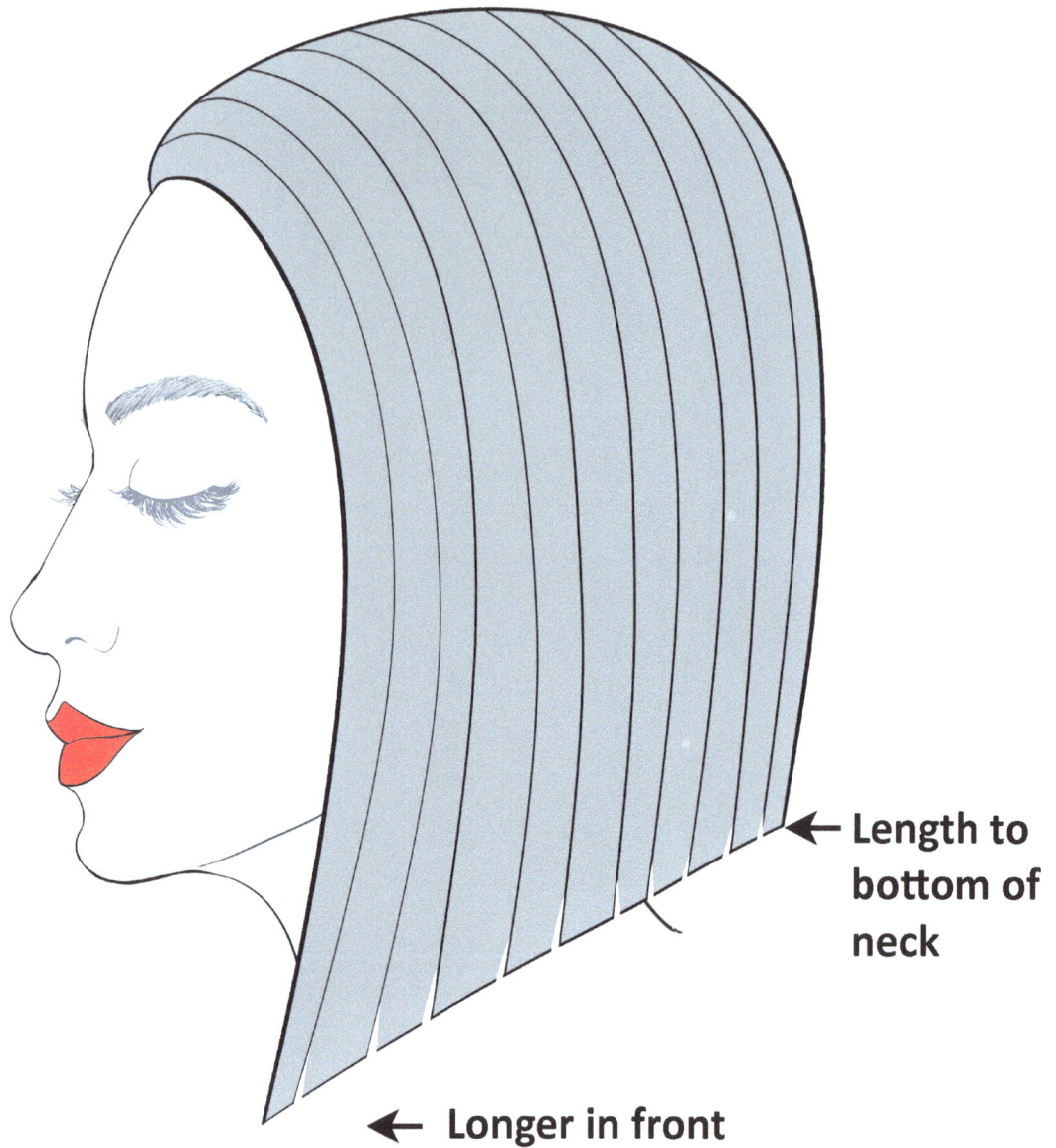

← Length to bottom of neck

← Longer in front

MEDIUM LENGTH - CENTER PART

THE A-LINE HAIRCUT

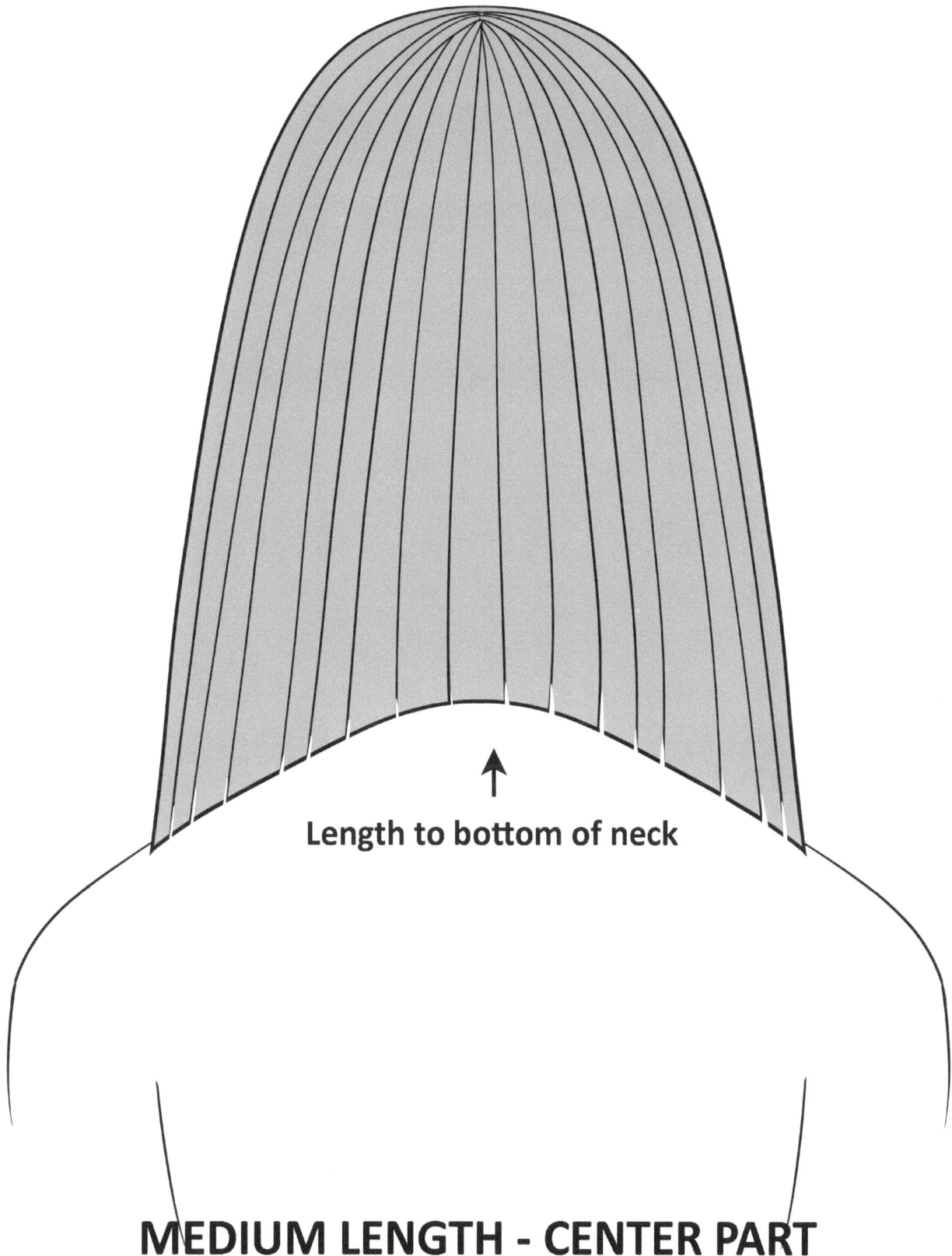

Length to bottom of neck

MEDIUM LENGTH - CENTER PART

THE A-LINE HAIRCUT

Disconnected Bang Options

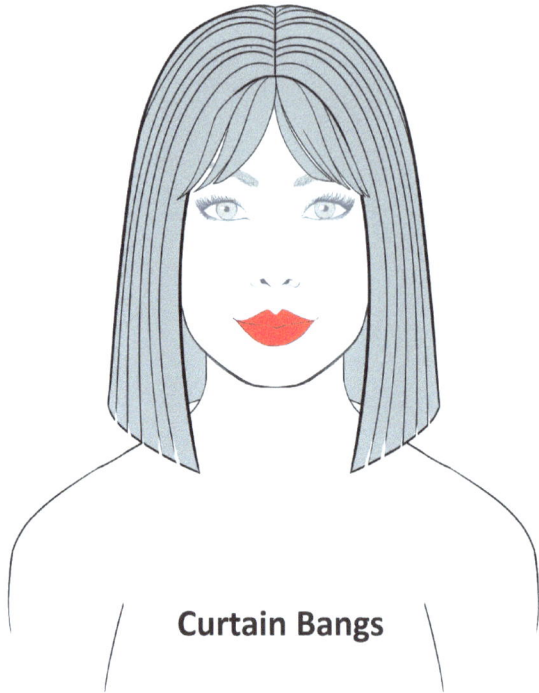

Curtain Bangs

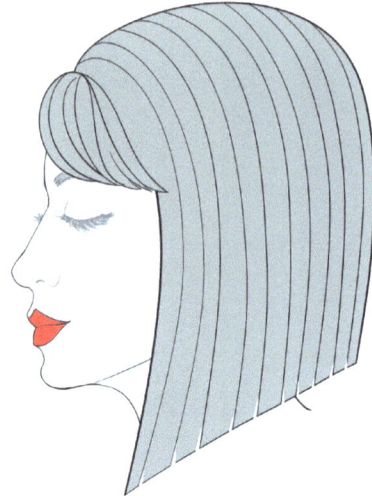

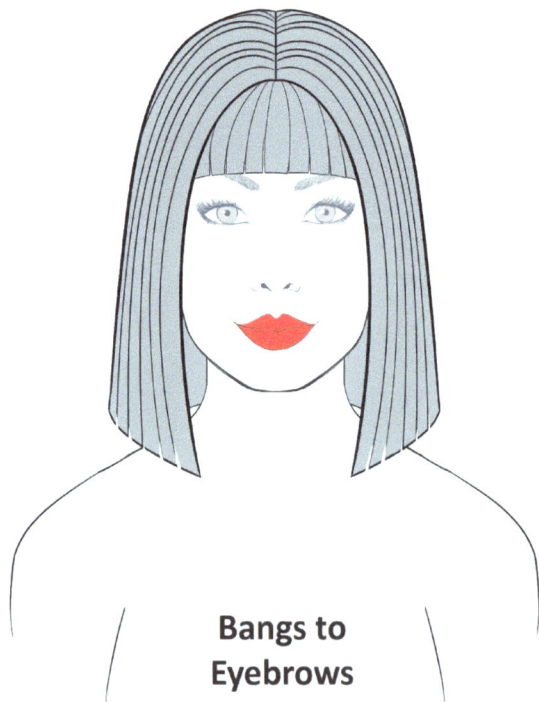

Curtain Bangs

Bangs to Eyebrows

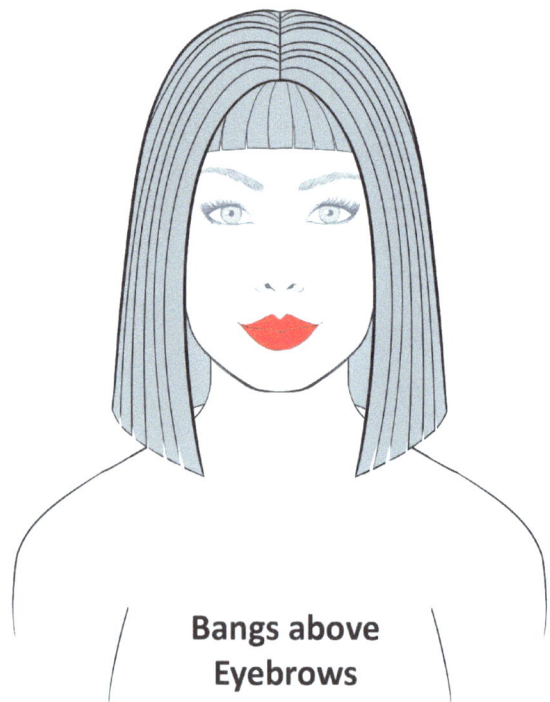

Bangs above Eyebrows

MEDIUM LENGTH - CENTER PART

THE A-LINE HAIRCUT

Curly Version

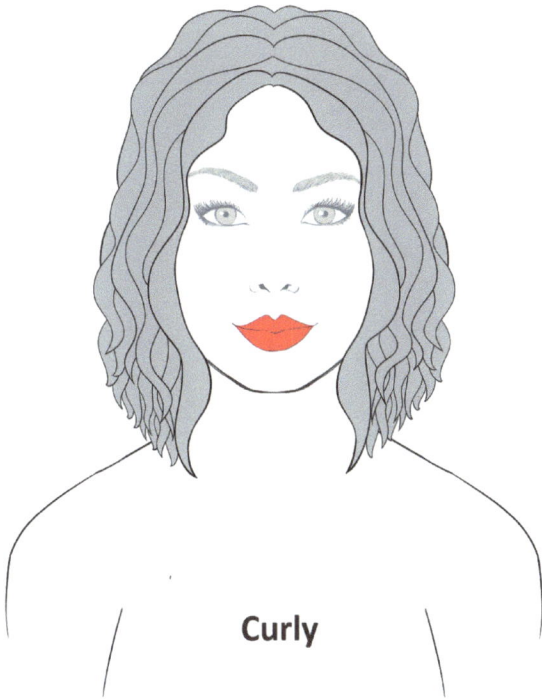

Curly

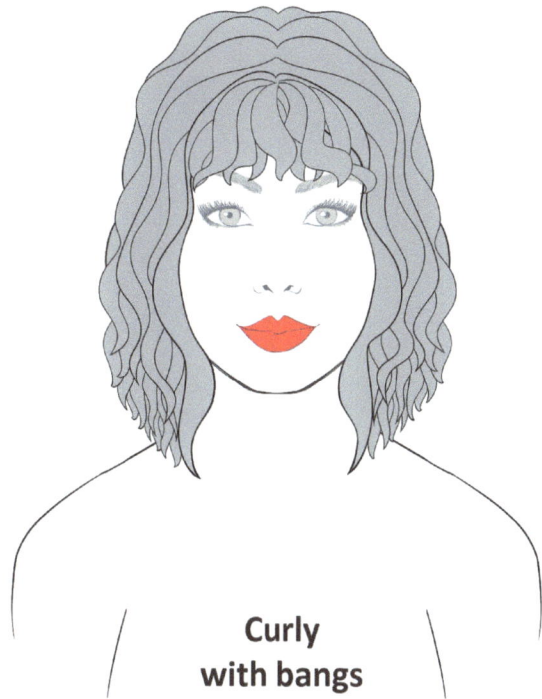

Curly
with bangs

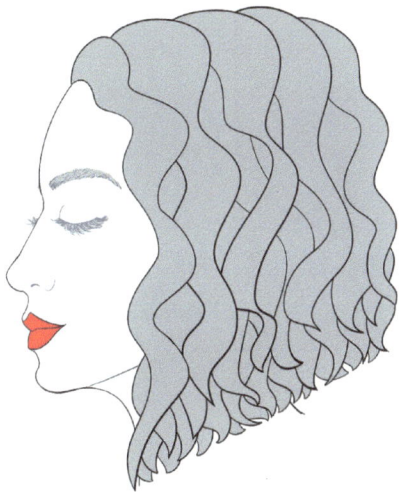

Curly

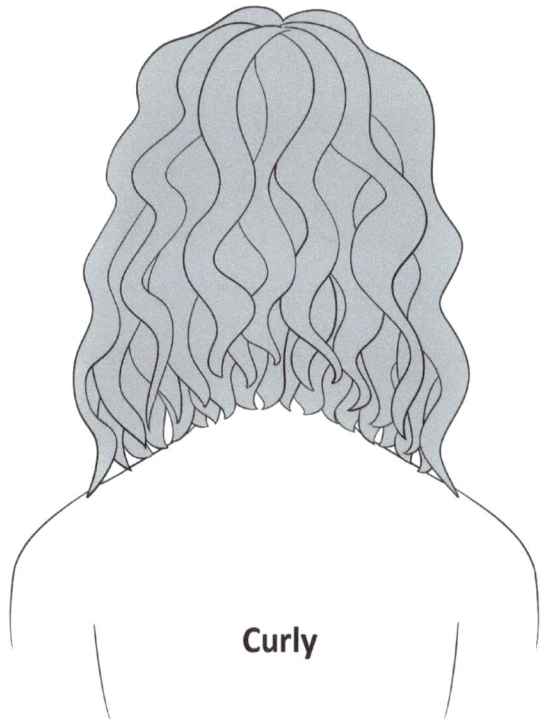

Curly

MEDIUM LENGTH - CENTER PART

THE A-LINE HAIRCUT

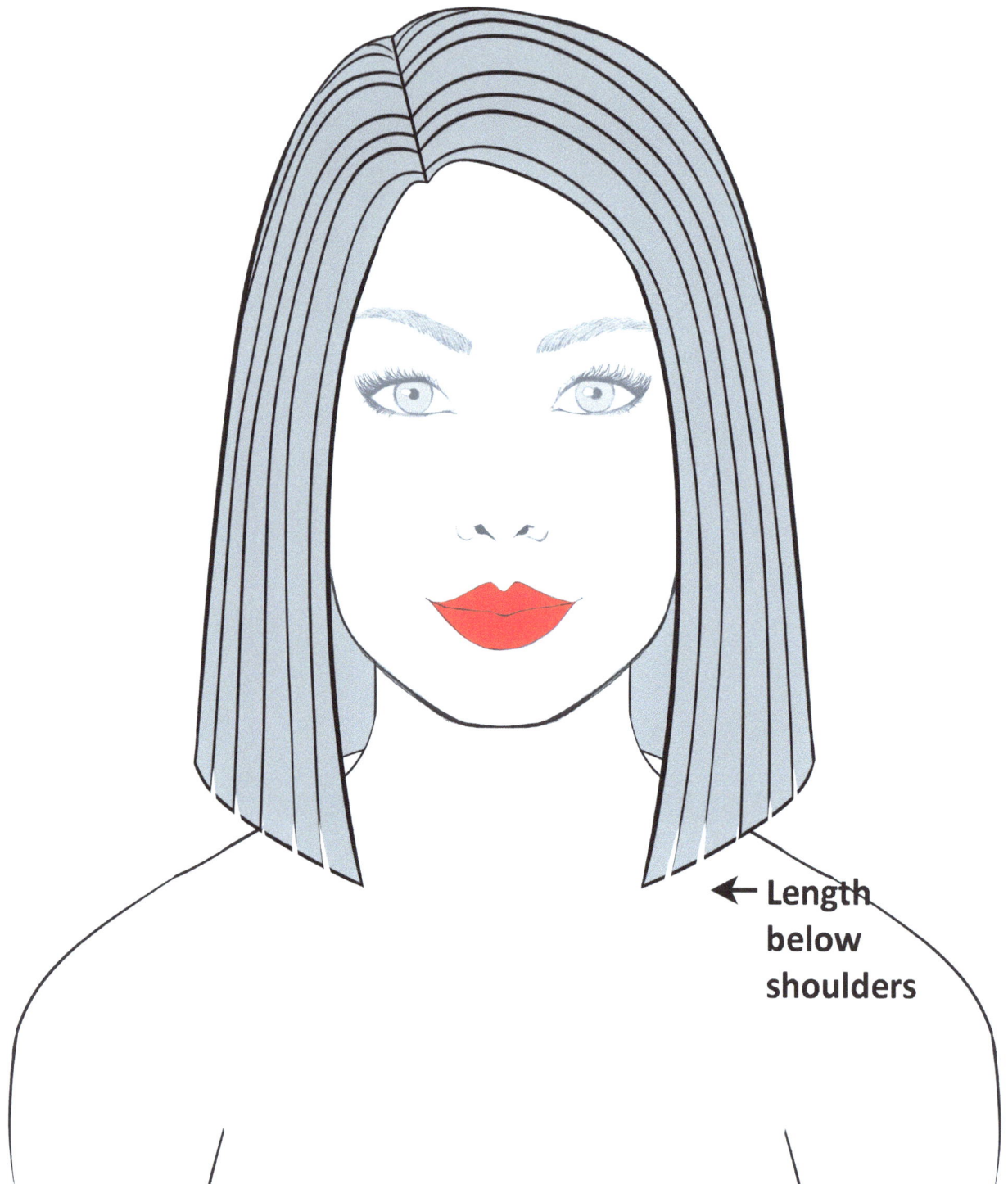

← **Length below shoulders**

MEDIUM LENGTH - SIDE PART

THE A-LINE HAIRCUT

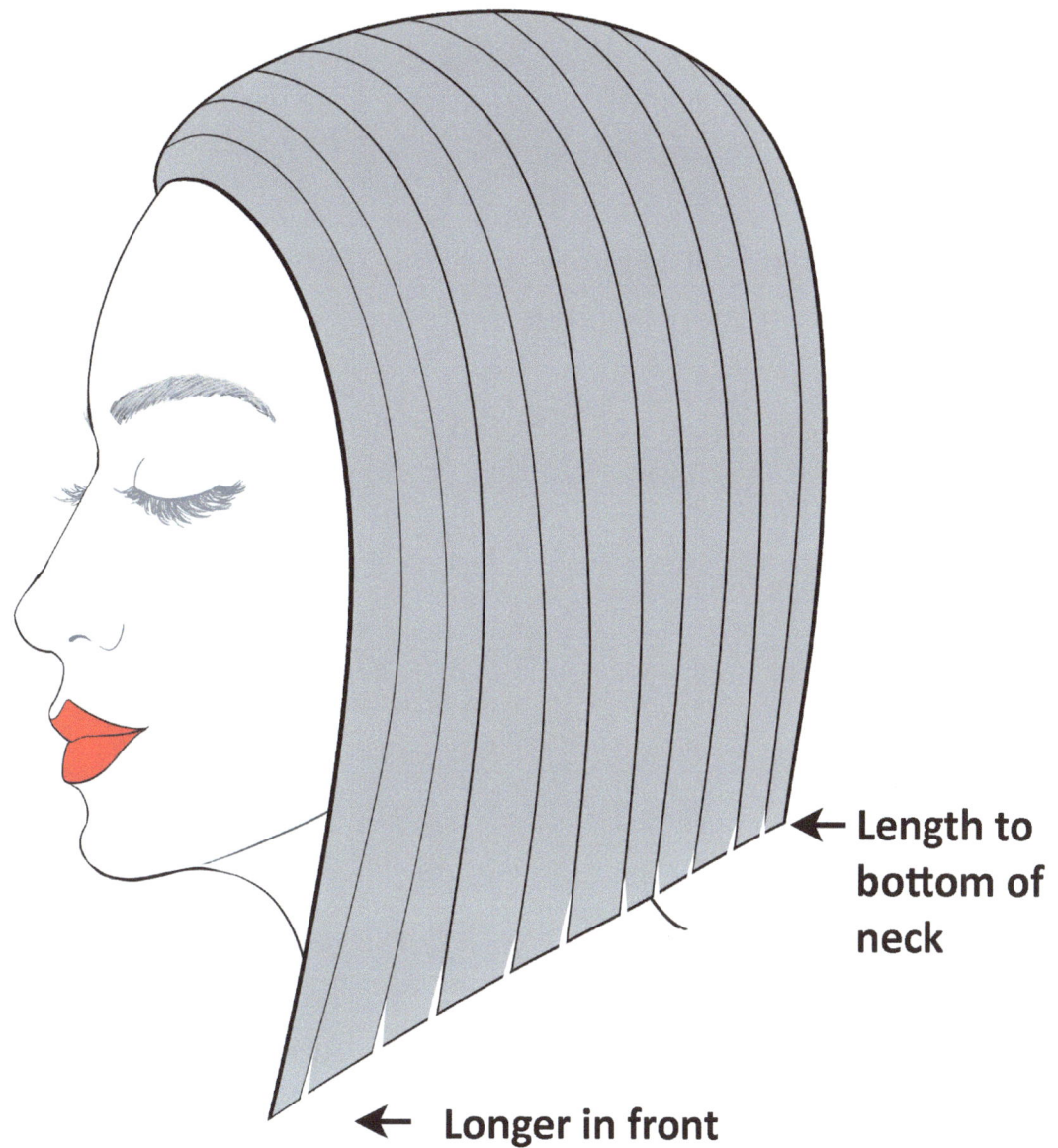

← Length to bottom of neck

← Longer in front

MEDIUM LENGTH - SIDE PART

THE A-LINE HAIRCUT

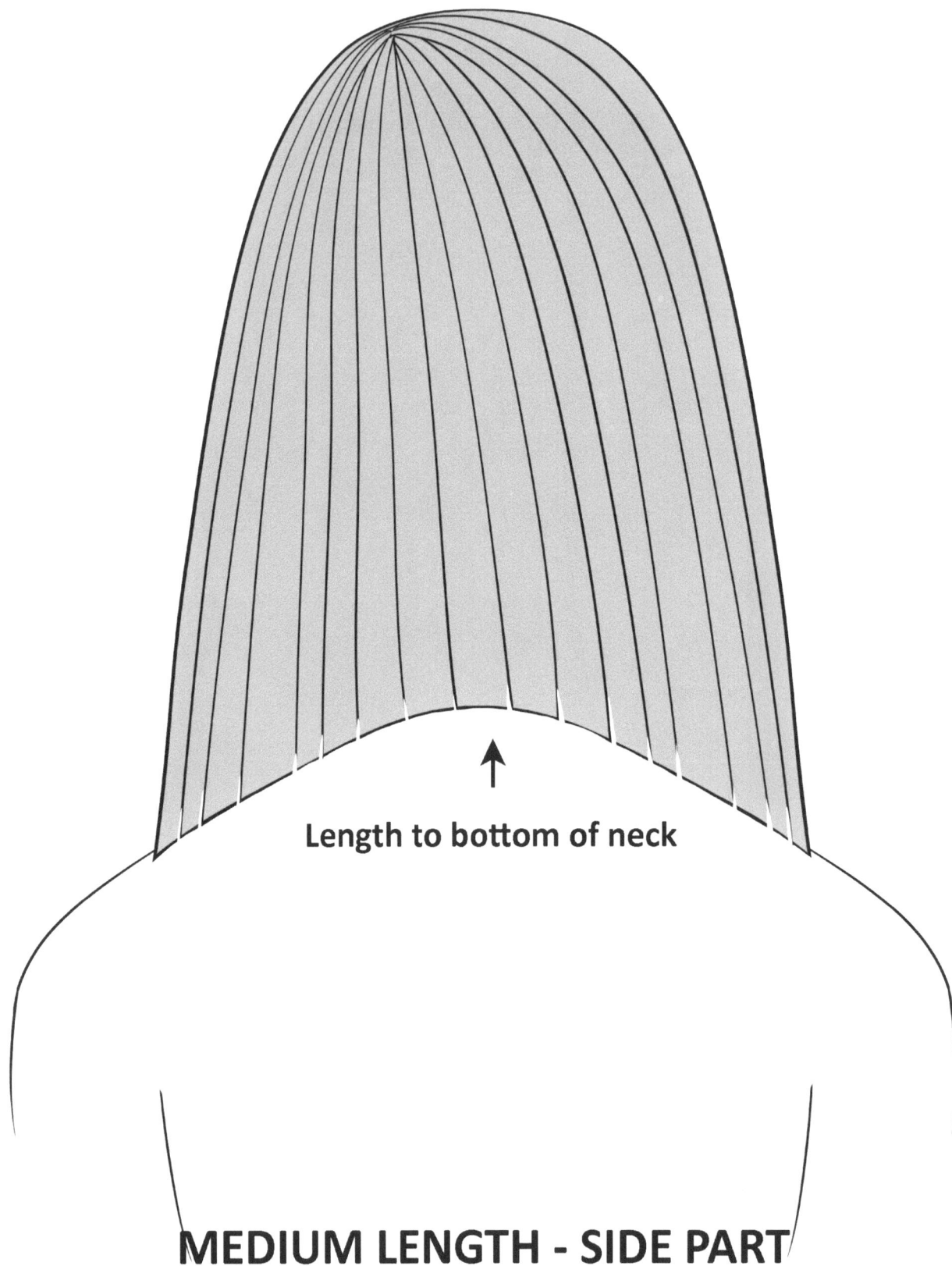

Length to bottom of neck

MEDIUM LENGTH - SIDE PART

THE A-LINE HAIRCUT

Disconnected Bang Options

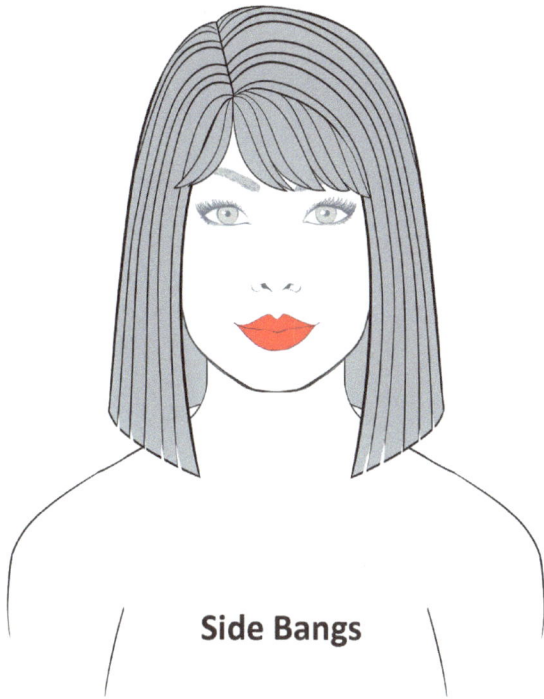

Side Bangs

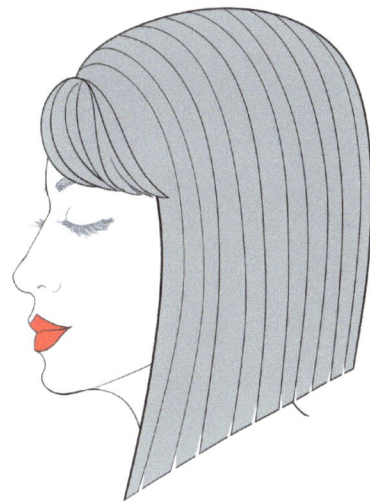

Side Bangs

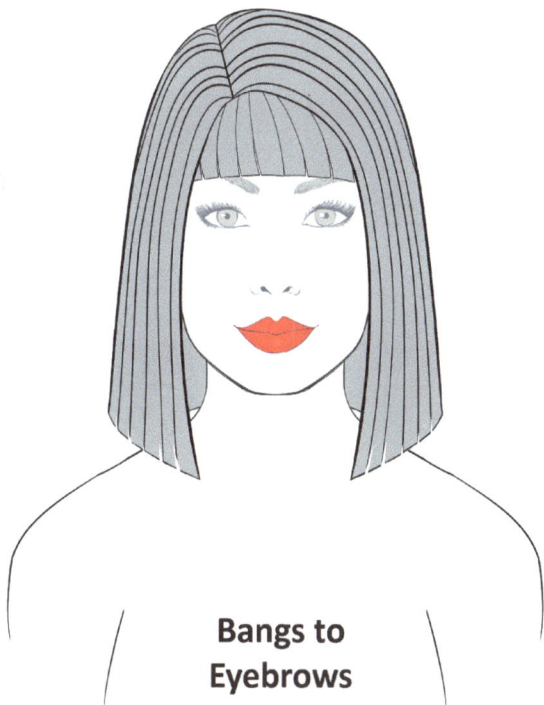

Bangs to Eyebrows

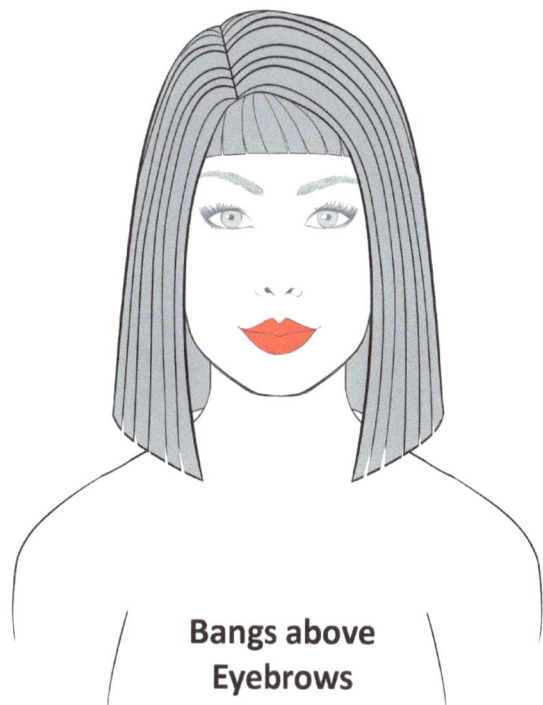

Bangs above Eyebrows

MEDIUM LENGTH - SIDE PART

THE A-LINE HAIRCUT

Curly Version

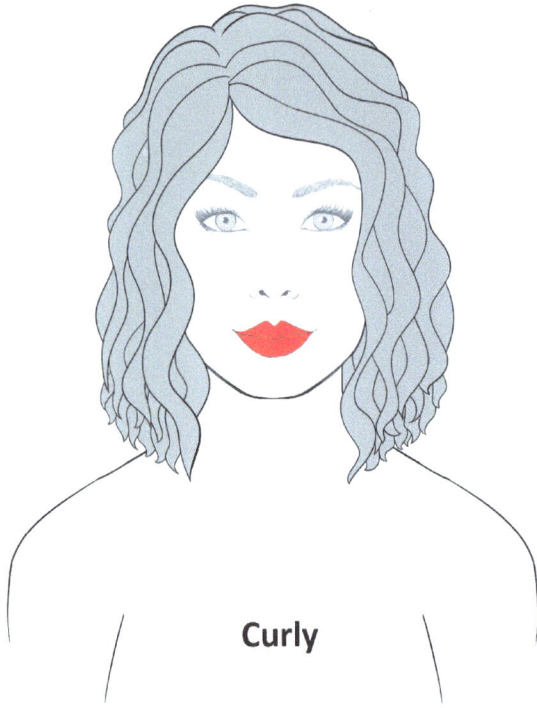

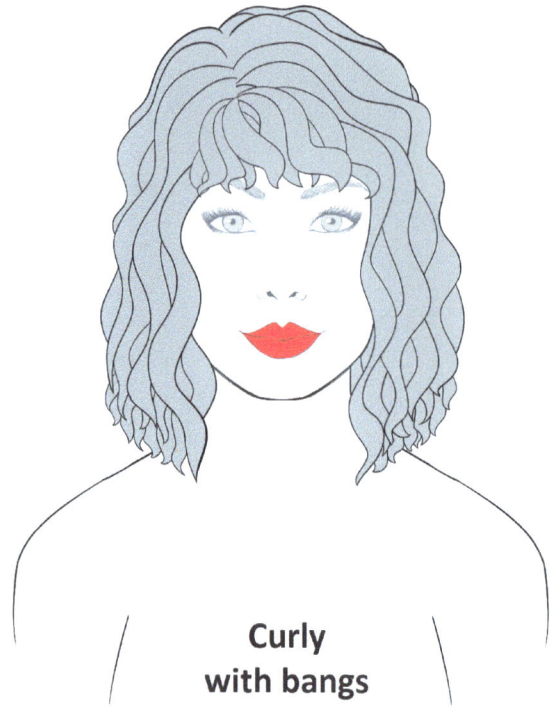

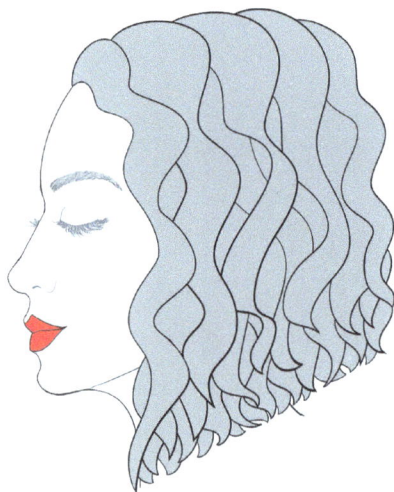

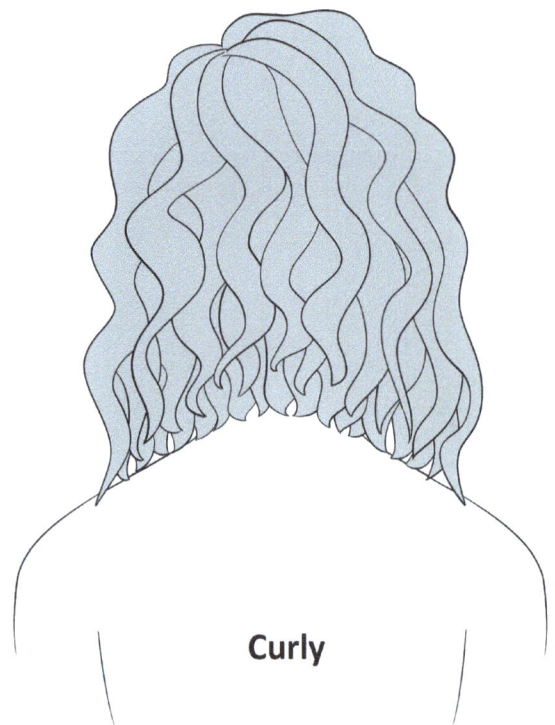

Curly

Curly
with bangs

Curly

Curly

MEDIUM LENGTH - SIDE PART

Chapter 4
THE BOB HAIRCUT

This sophisticated haircut offers timeless beauty and is easy to maintain.

- **LENGTH-** The Bob Haircut looks great in short lengths and medium lengths.

- **PART-** This haircut has a fixed part and is not interchangeable.

- **BANGS-** Looks great with or without bangs.

- **LAYERS-** Choose light layers or no layers to serve your unique hair texture and hair type.

- **STYLING-** The Bob Haircut is a breeze to style. Simply blow dry and if needed use a flat iron for a polished look.

THE BOB HAIRCUT

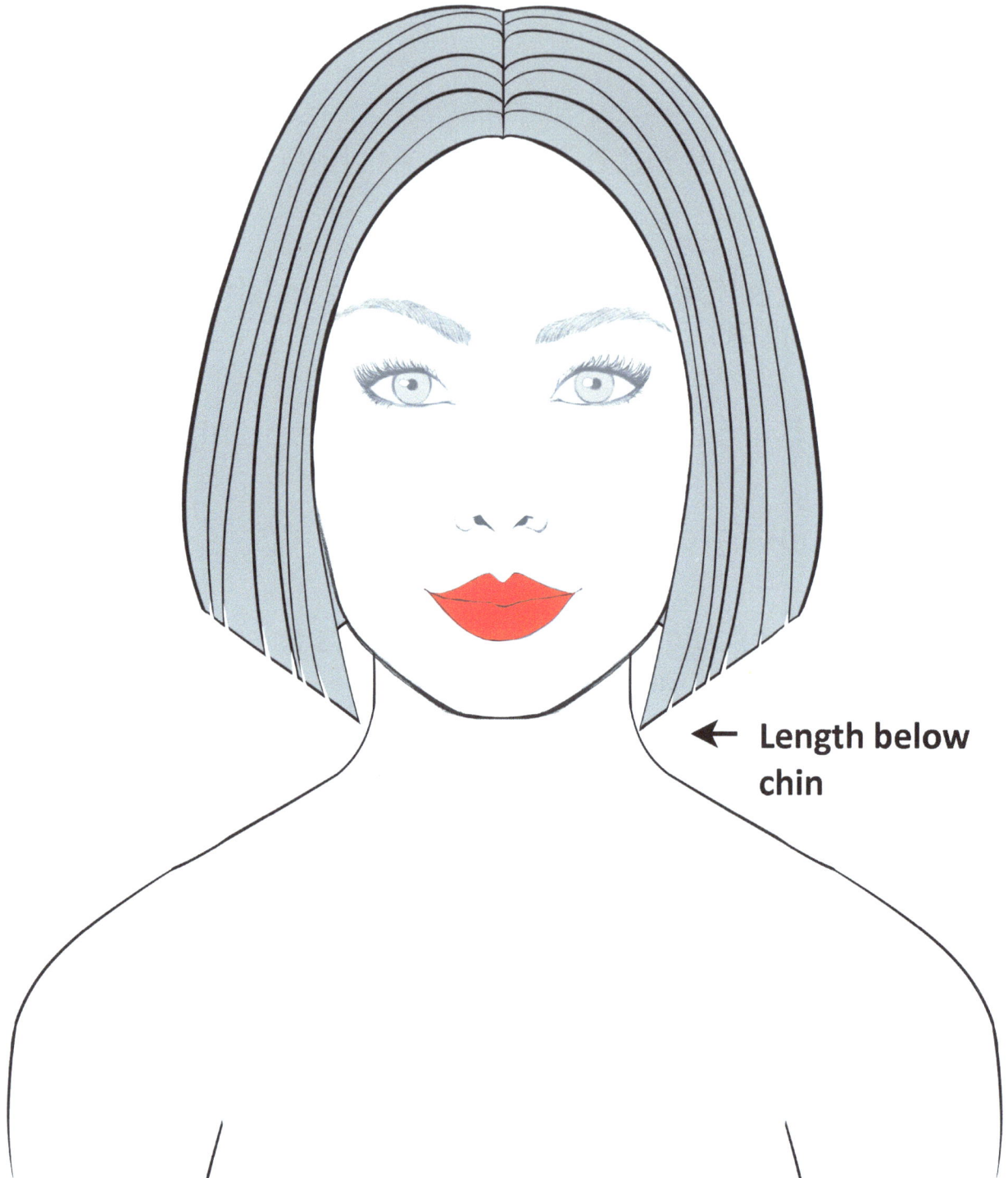

← Length below chin

SHORT LENGTH - CENTER PART

THE BOB HAIRCUT

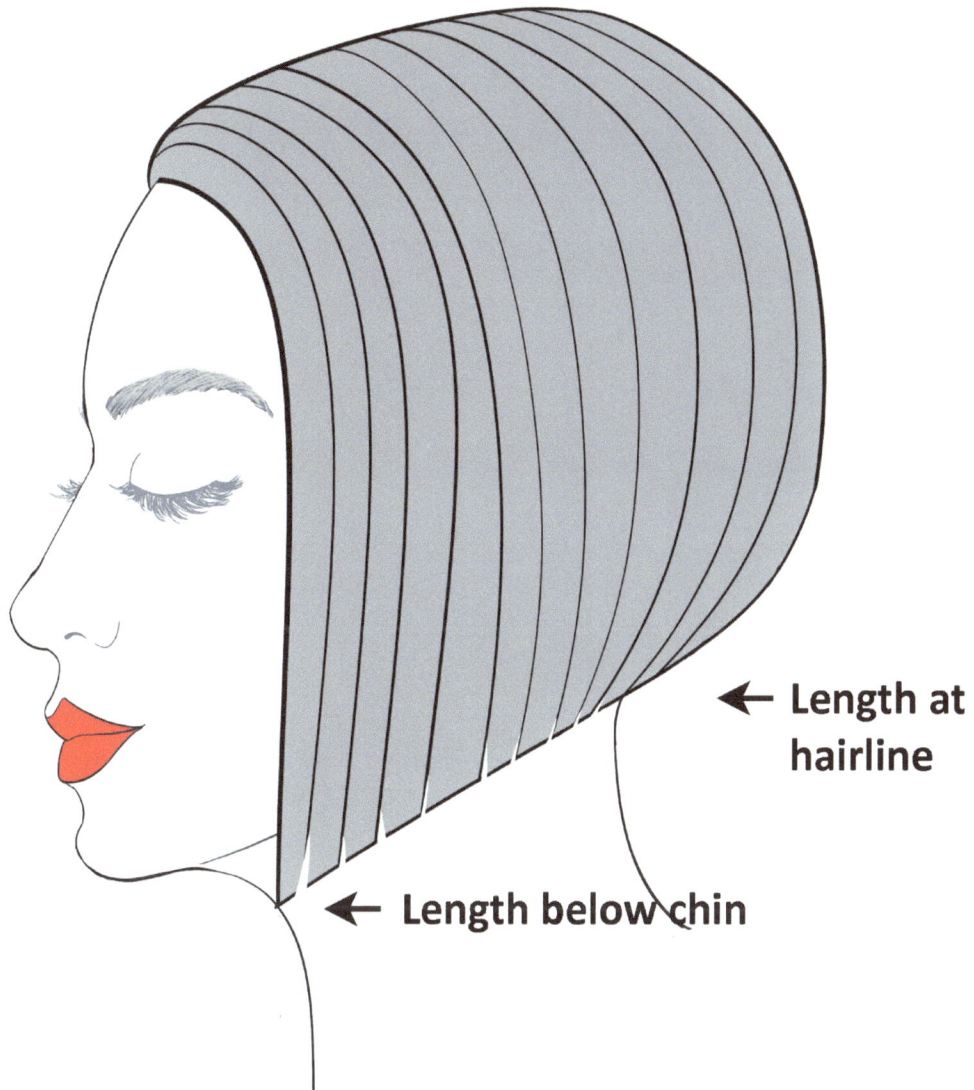

← **Length at hairline**

← **Length below chin**

SHORT LENGTH - CENTER PART

THE BOB HAIRCUT

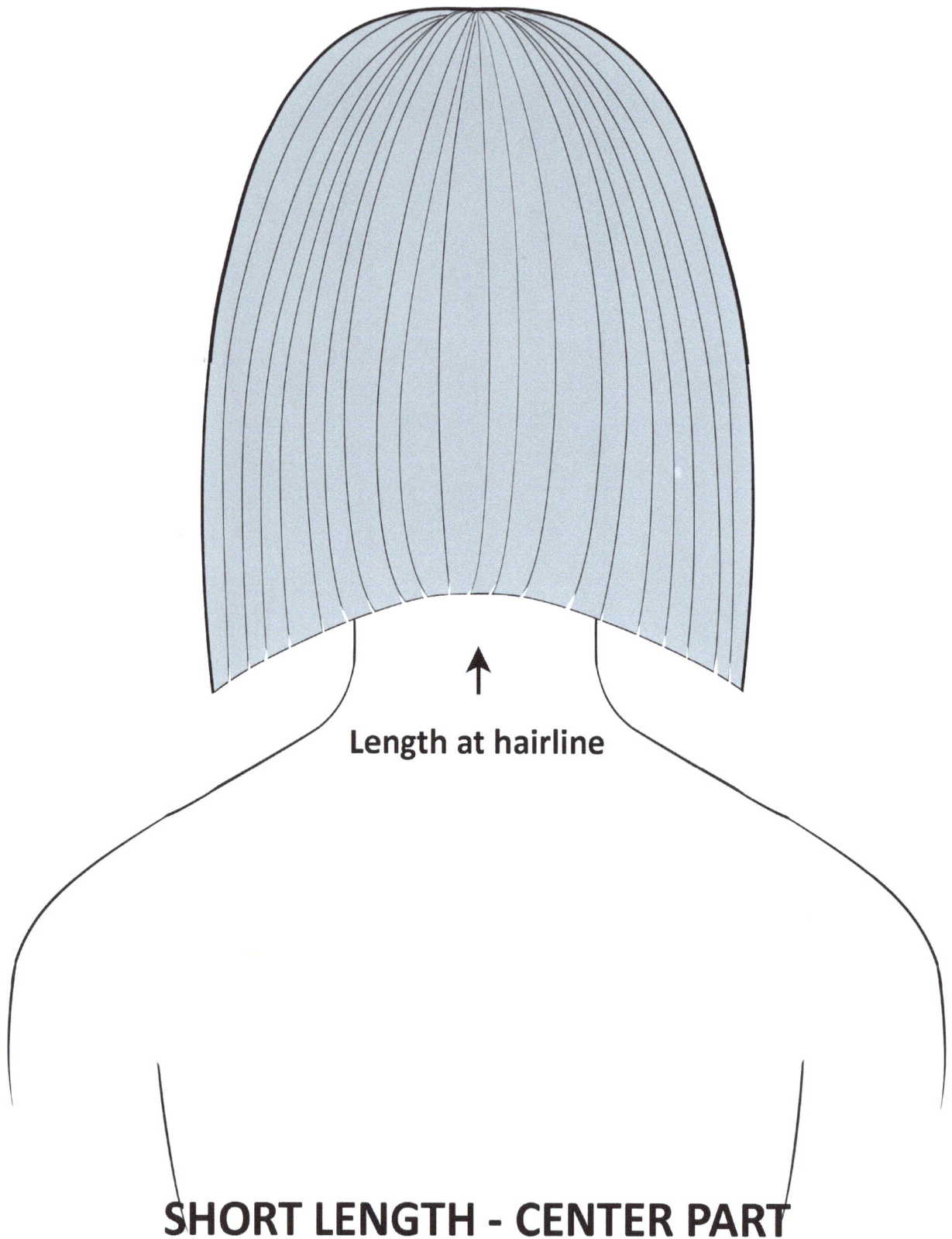

Length at hairline

SHORT LENGTH - CENTER PART

THE BOB HAIRCUT

Disconnected Bang Options

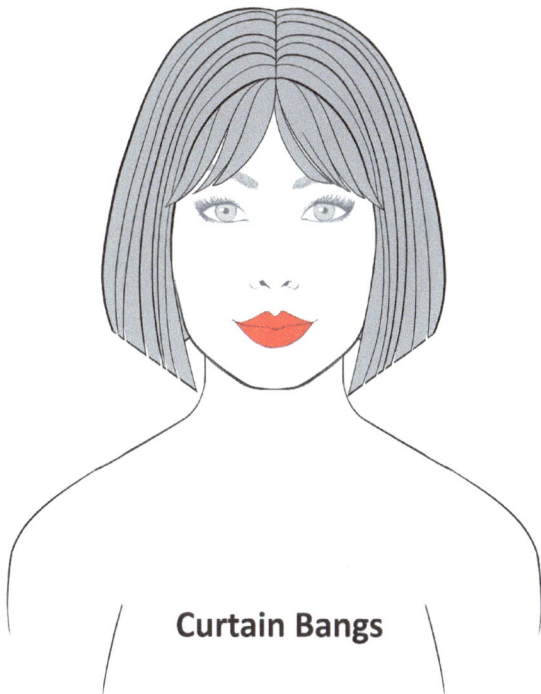

Curtain Bangs

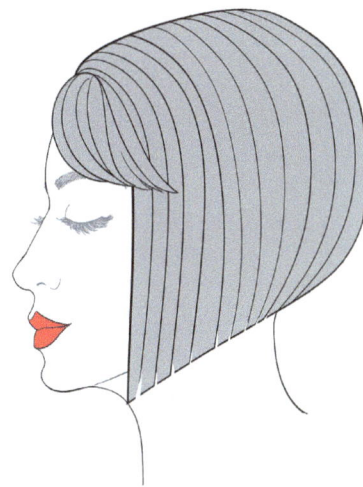

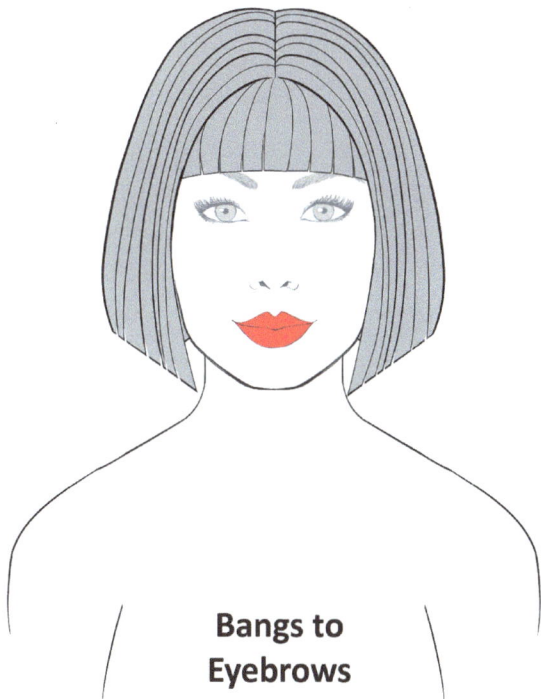

Curtain Bangs

Bangs to
Eyebrows

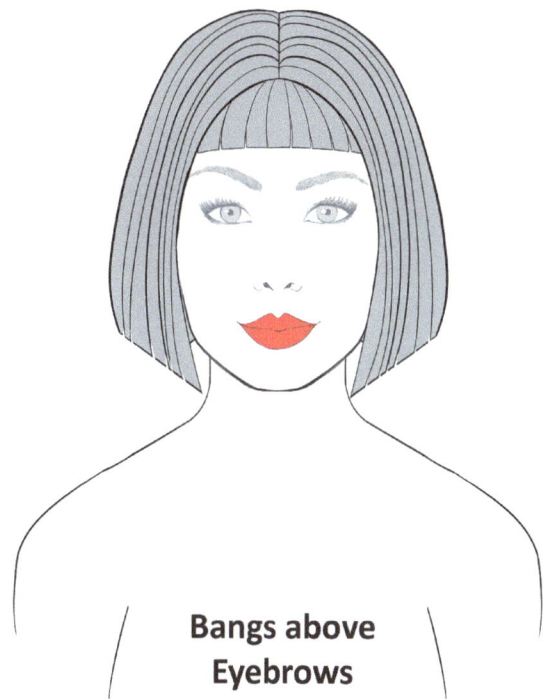

Bangs above
Eyebrows

SHORT LENGTH - CENTER PART

THE BOB HAIRCUT

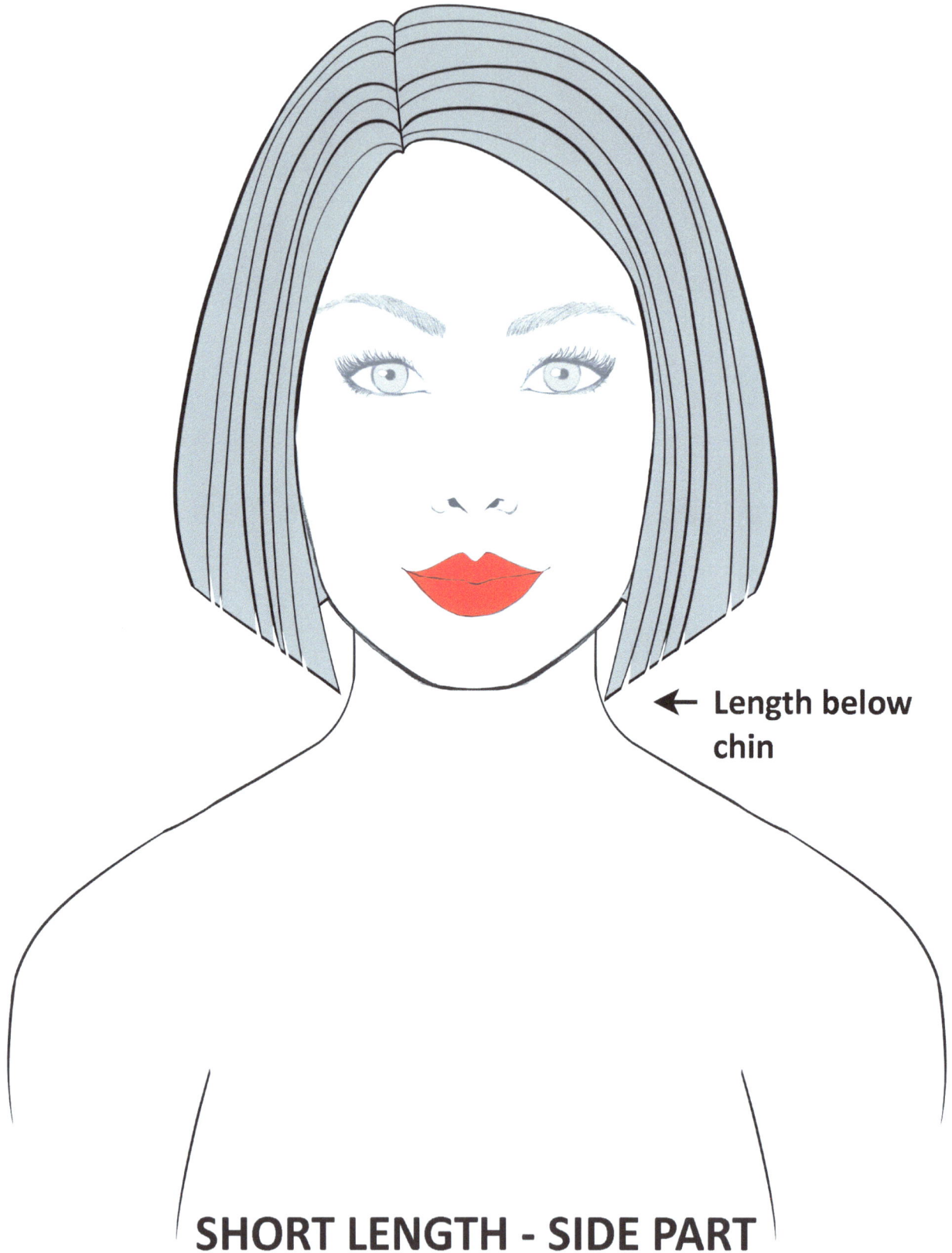

← **Length below chin**

SHORT LENGTH - SIDE PART

THE BOB HAIRCUT

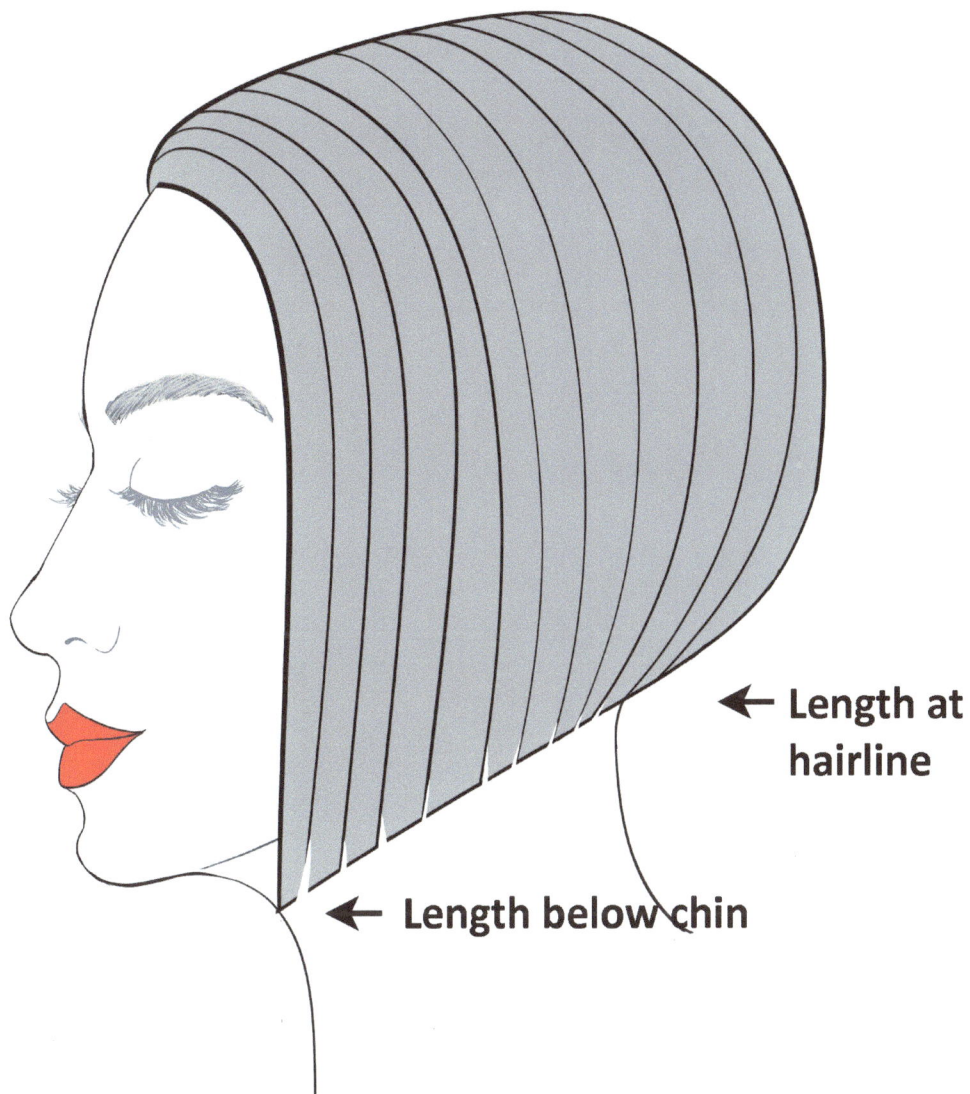

← Length at
   hairline

← Length below chin

SHORT LENGTH - SIDE PART

THE BOB HAIRCUT

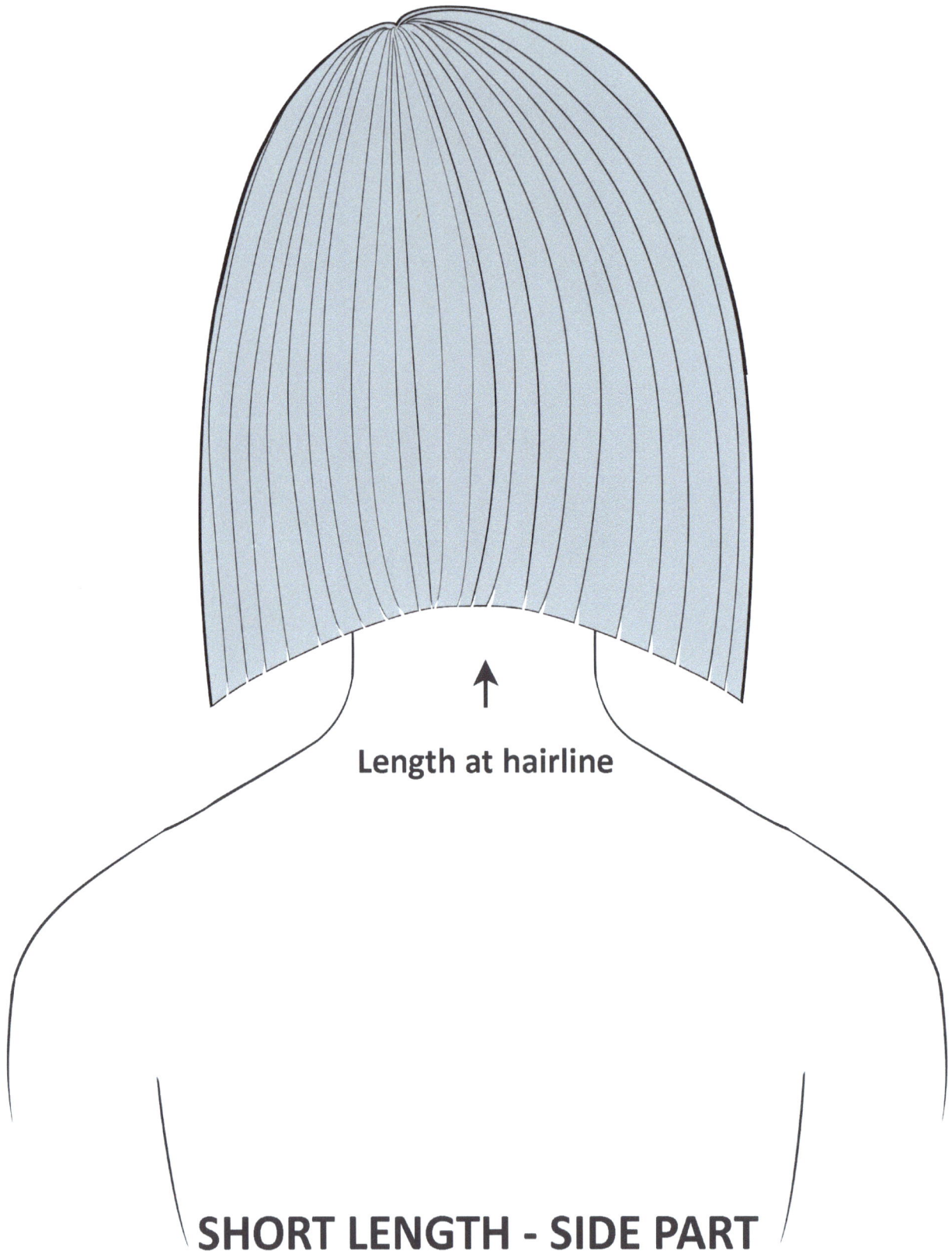

Length at hairline

SHORT LENGTH - SIDE PART

THE BOB HAIRCUT

Disconnected Bang Options

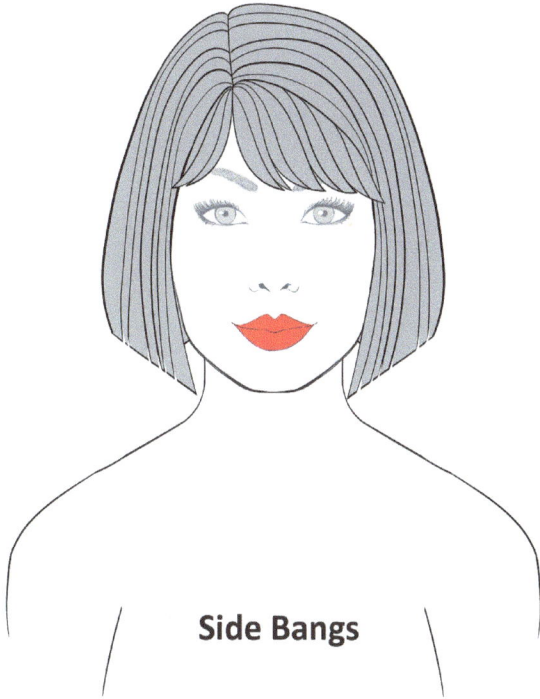

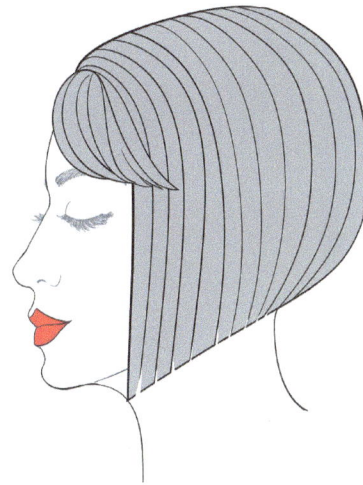

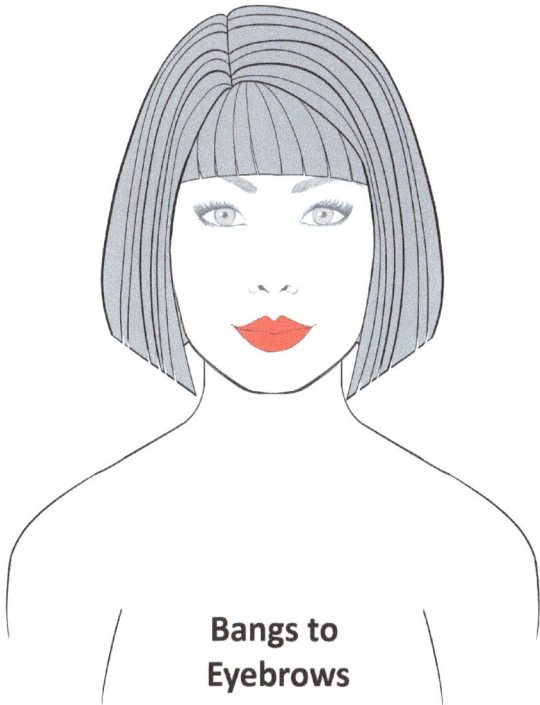

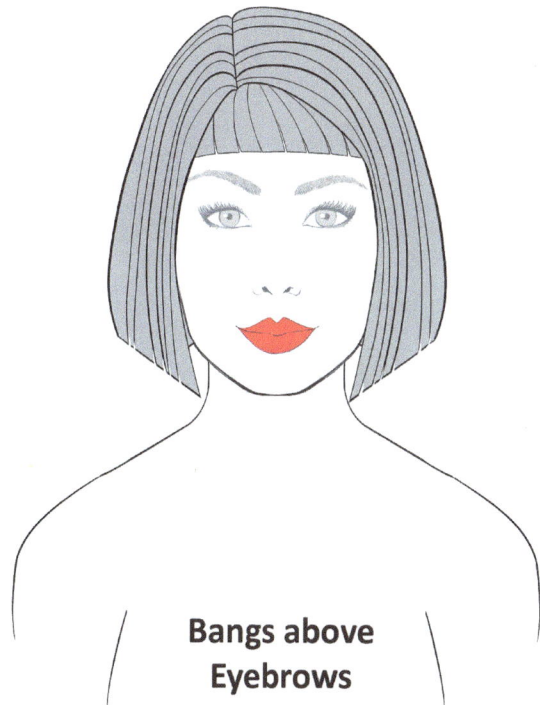

Side Bangs

Side Bangs

Bangs to
Eyebrows

Bangs above
Eyebrows

SHORT LENGTH - SIDE PART

THE BOB HAIRCUT

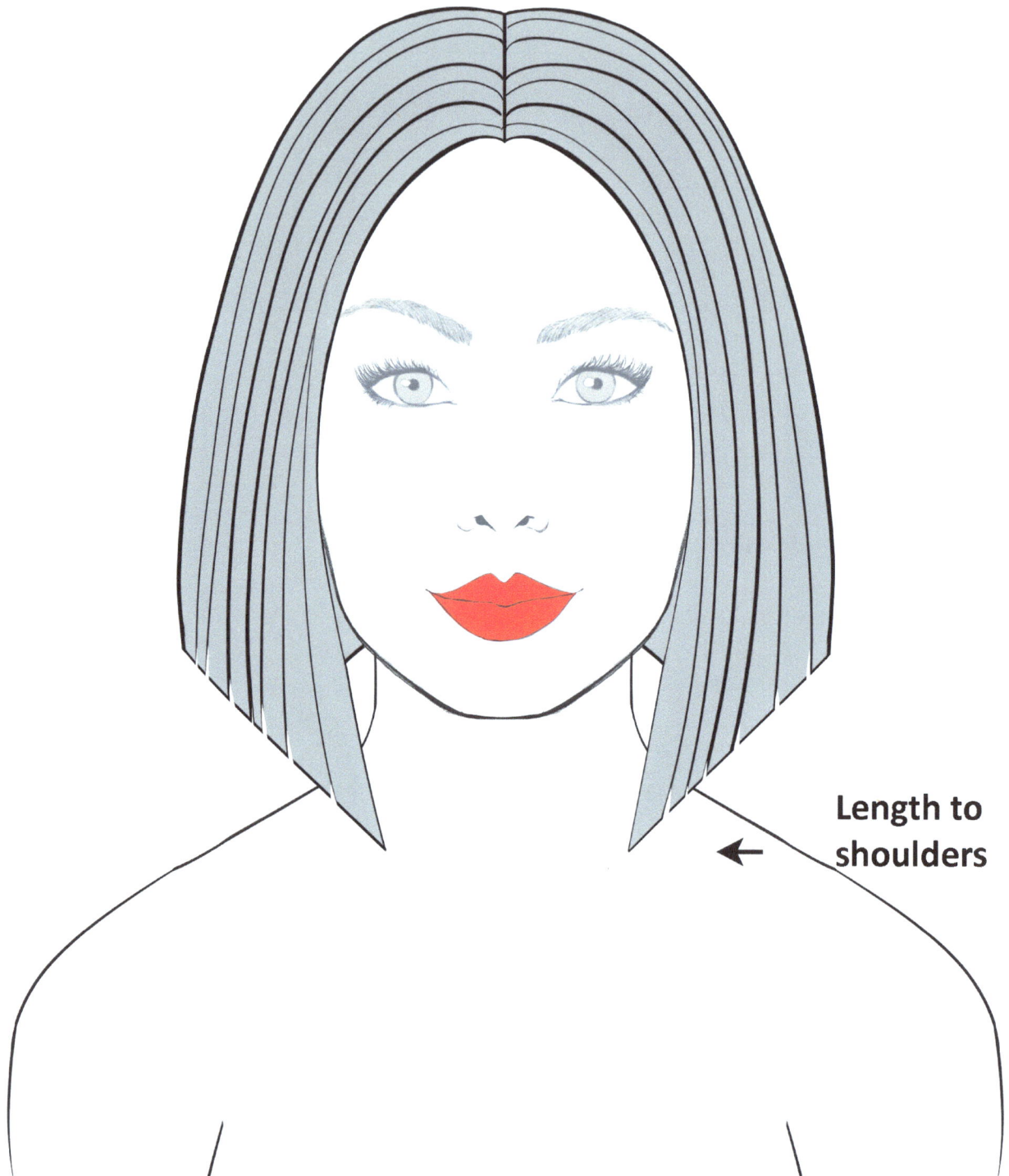

Length to shoulders

MEDIUM LENGTH - CENTER PART

THE BOB HAIRCUT

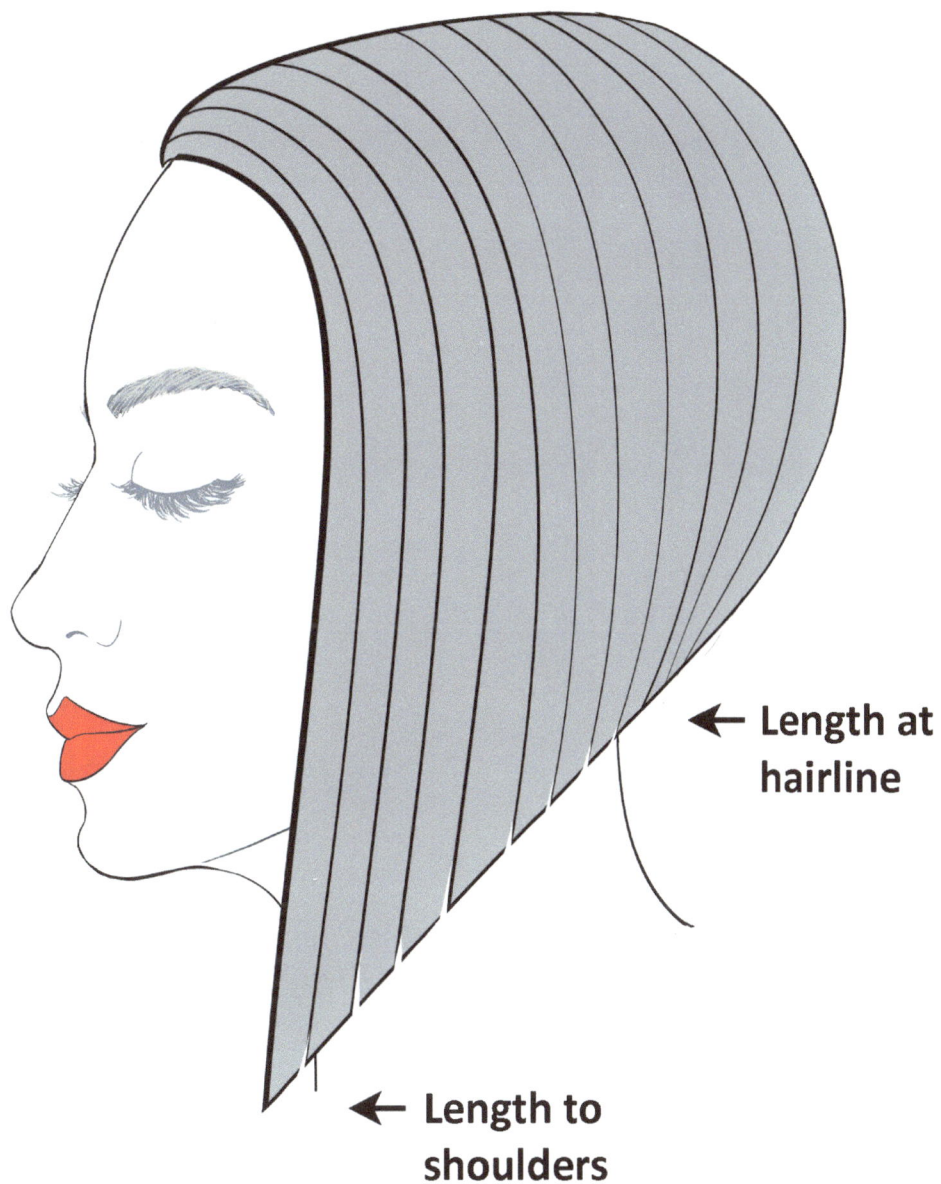

← **Length at hairline**

← **Length to shoulders**

MEDIUM LENGTH - CENTER PART

THE BOB HAIRCUT

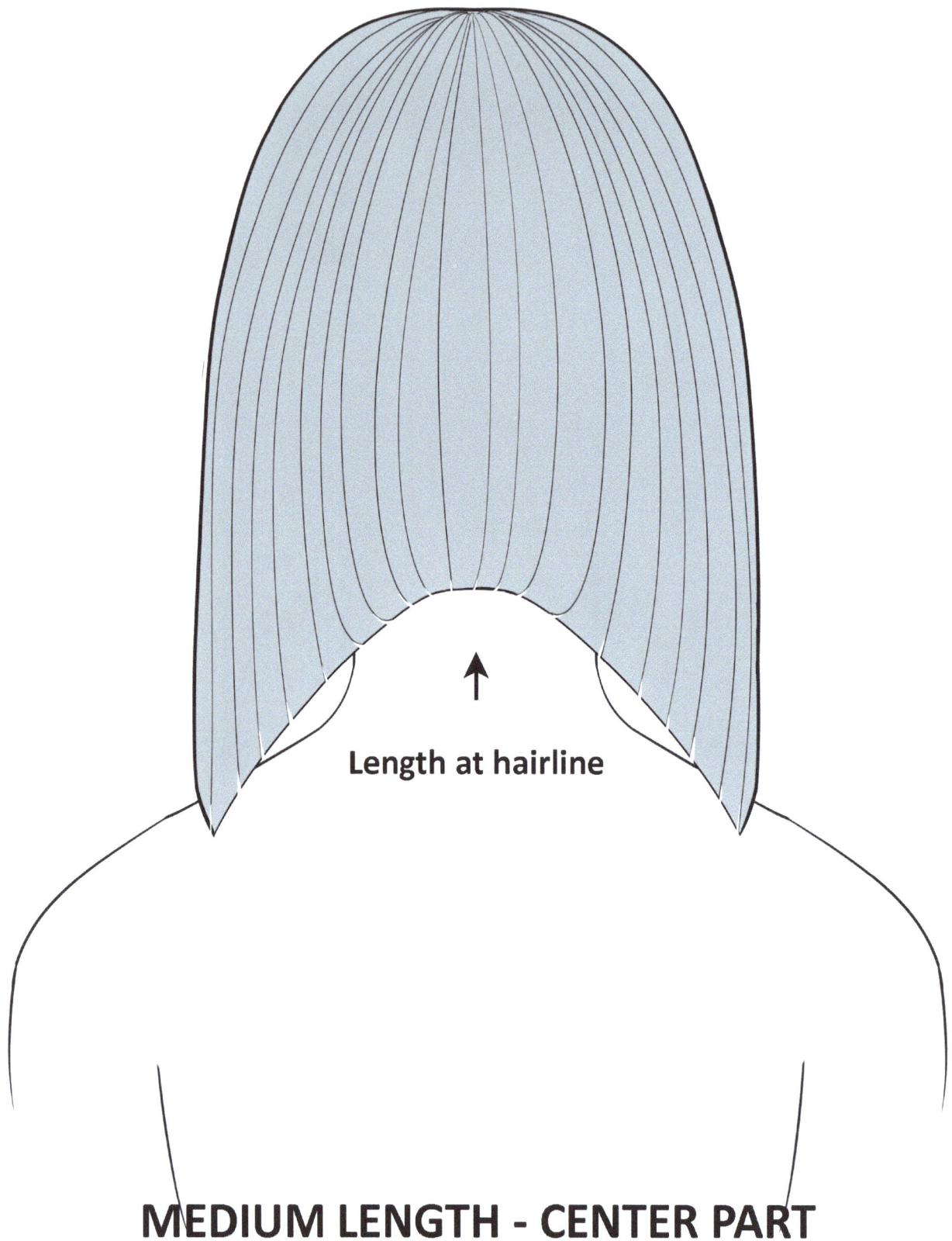

Length at hairline

MEDIUM LENGTH - CENTER PART

THE BOB HAIRCUT

Disconnected Bang Options

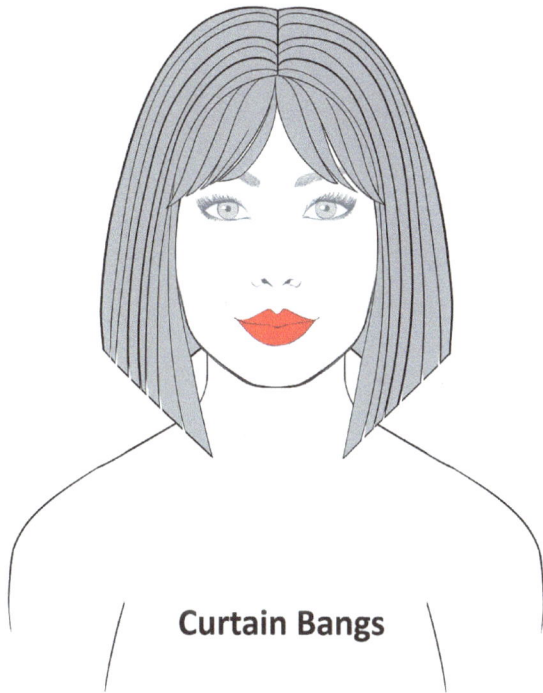

Curtain Bangs

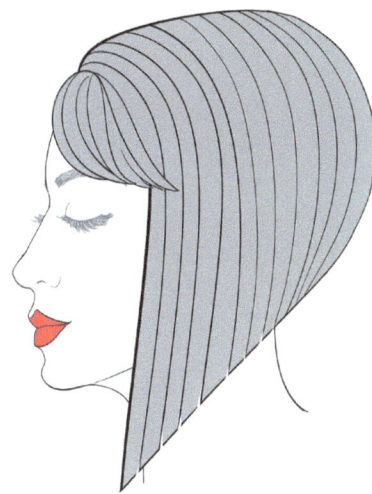

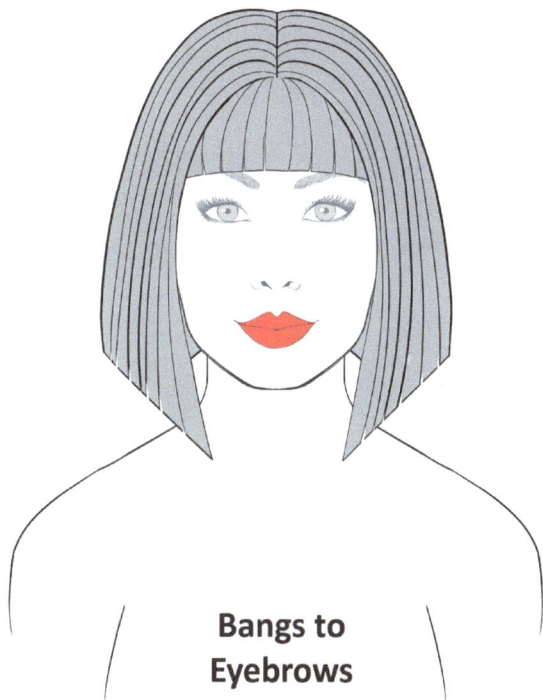

Curtain Bangs

Bangs to Eyebrows

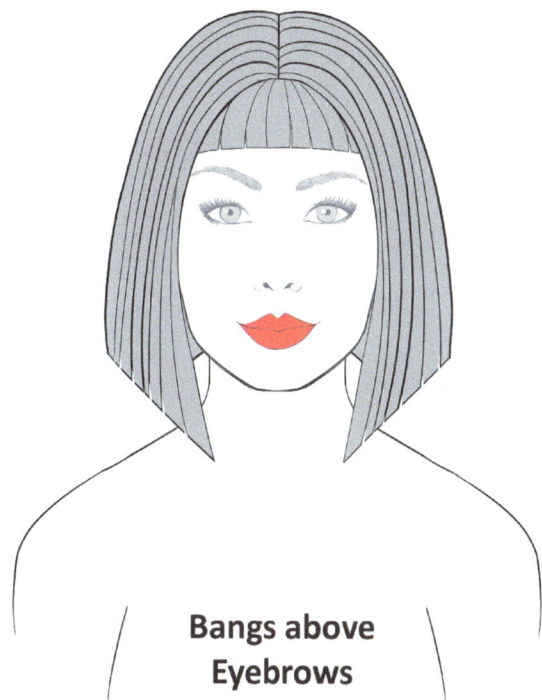

Bangs above Eyebrows

MEDIUM LENGTH - CENTER PART

THE BOB HAIRCUT

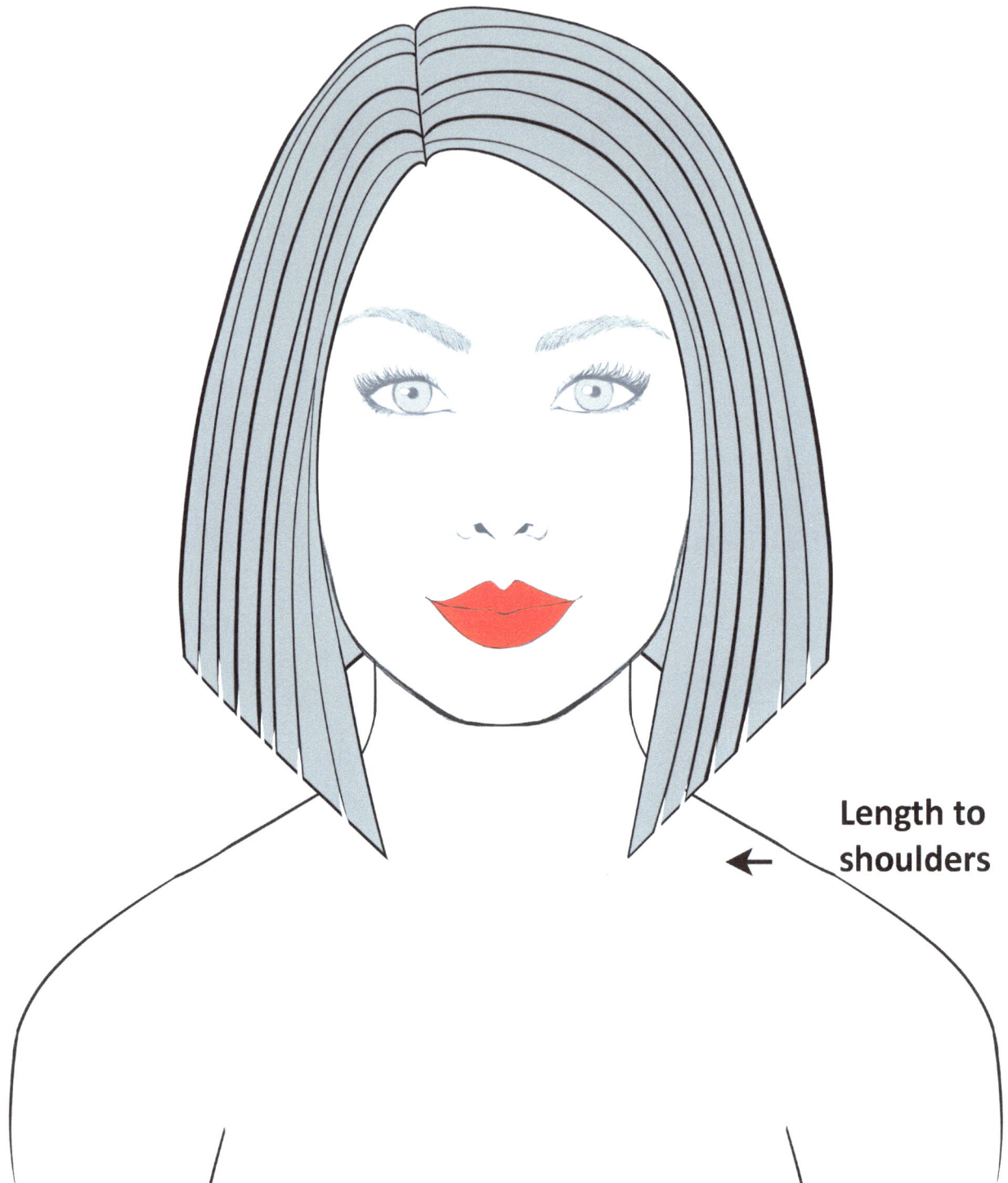

Length to
shoulders

MEDIUM LENGTH - SIDE PART

THE BOB HAIRCUT

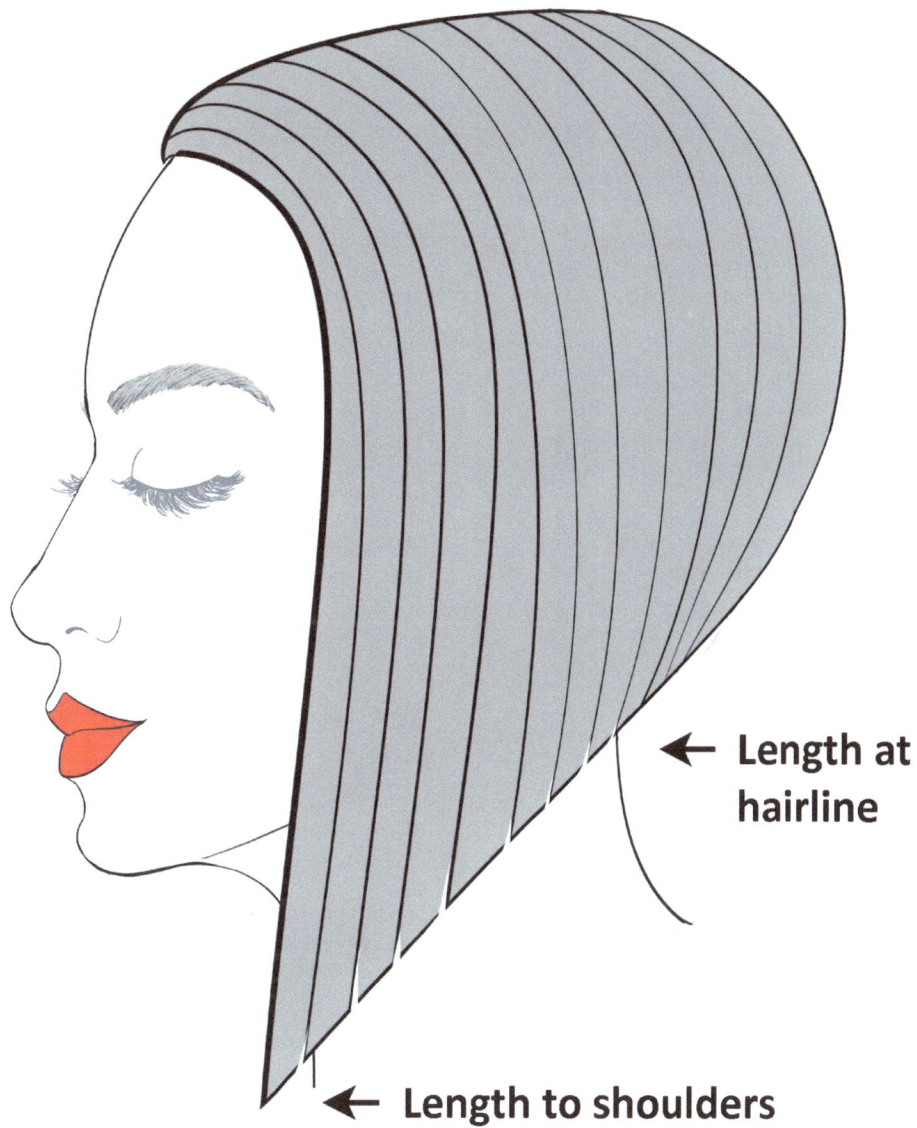

← Length at hairline

← Length to shoulders

MEDIUM LENGTH - SIDE PART

THE BOB HAIRCUT

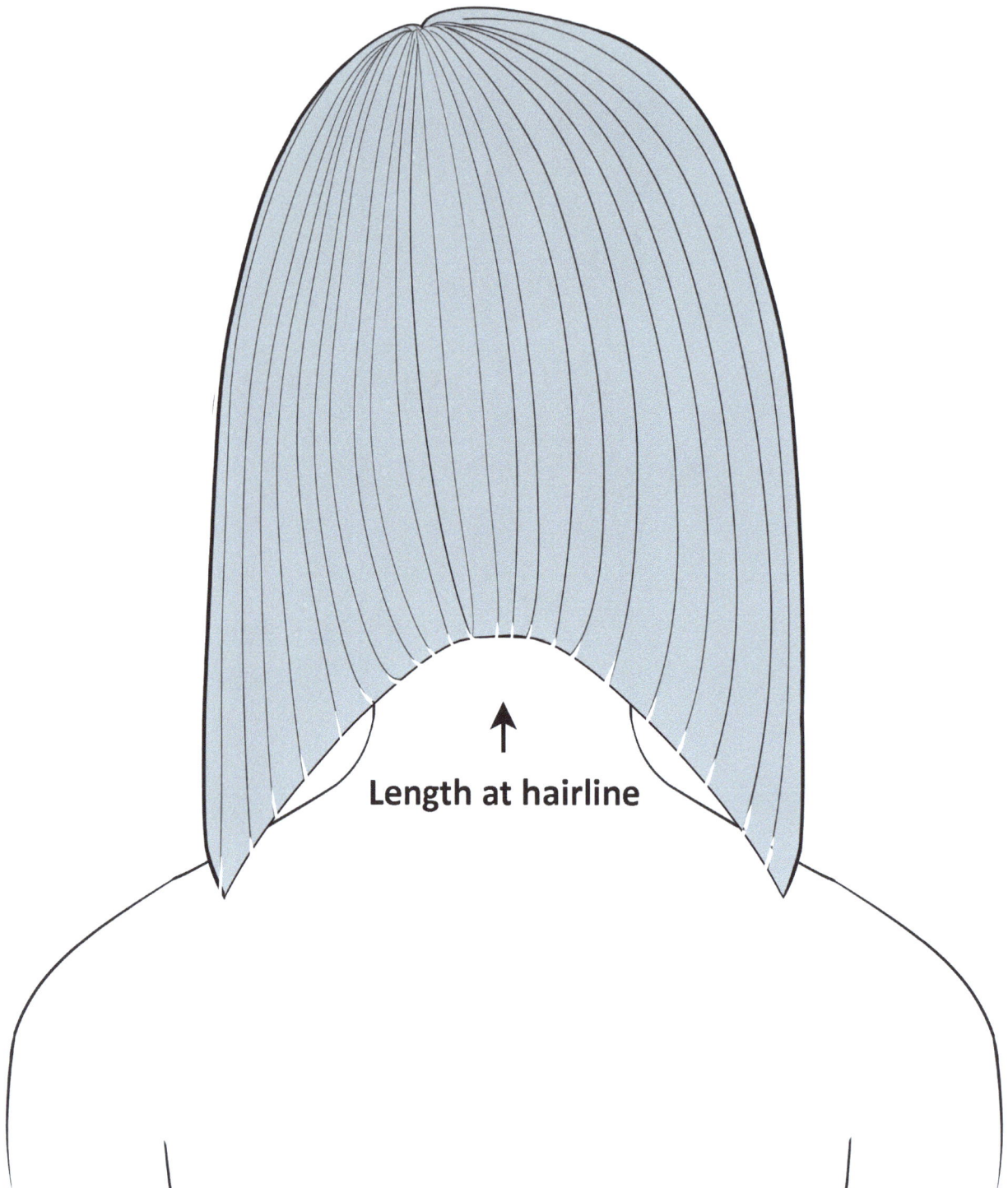

Length at hairline

MEDIUM LENGTH - SIDE PART

THE BOB HAIRCUT

Disconnected Bang Options

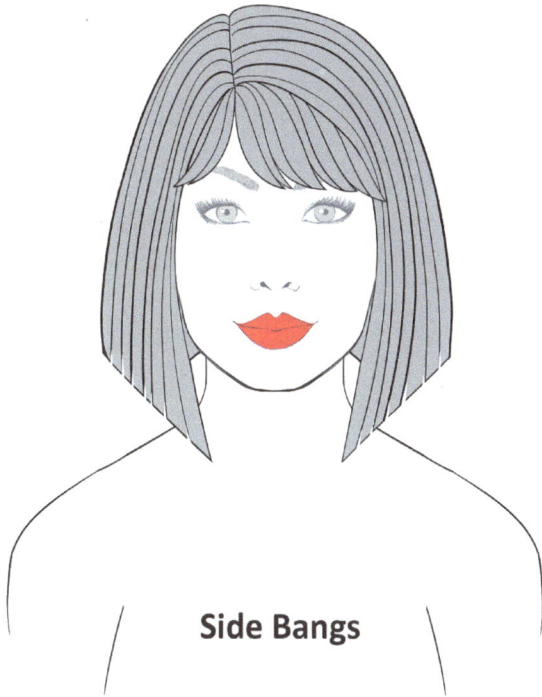

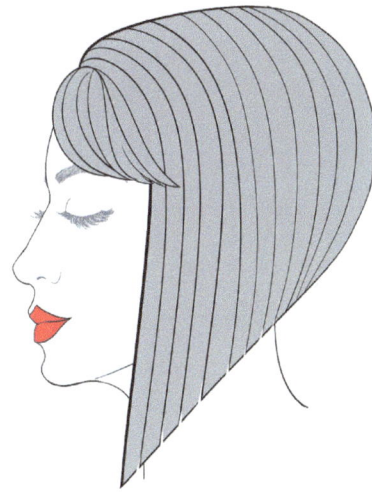

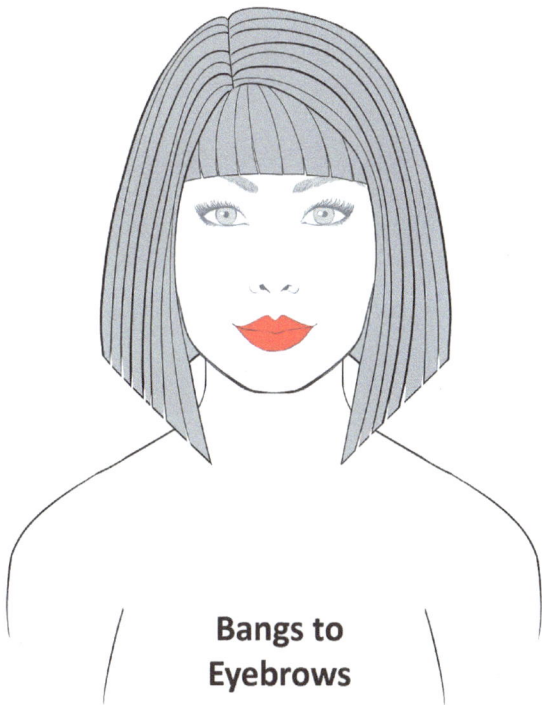

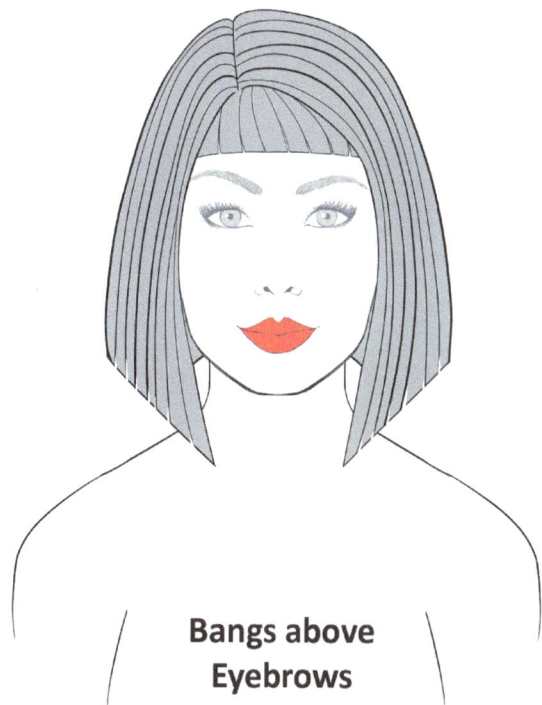

Side Bangs

Side Bangs

Bangs to Eyebrows

Bangs above Eyebrows

MEDIUM LENGTH - SIDE PART

Chapter 5
THE INVERTED BOB HAIRCUT

This edgy yet sophisticated haircut offers timeless beauty with a little spunk.

- **LENGTH-** The Inverted Bob Haircut looks great in short lengths and medium lengths.

- **PART-** This haircut has a fixed part and is not interchangeable.

- **BANGS-** Looks great with or without bangs.

- **LAYERS-** Choose light layers or no layers to serve your unique hair texture and hair type.

- **STYLING-** The Inverted Bob Haircut is quick and easy to style. Simply blow dry and if needed use a flat iron for a polished finish.

THE INVERTED BOB HAIRCUT

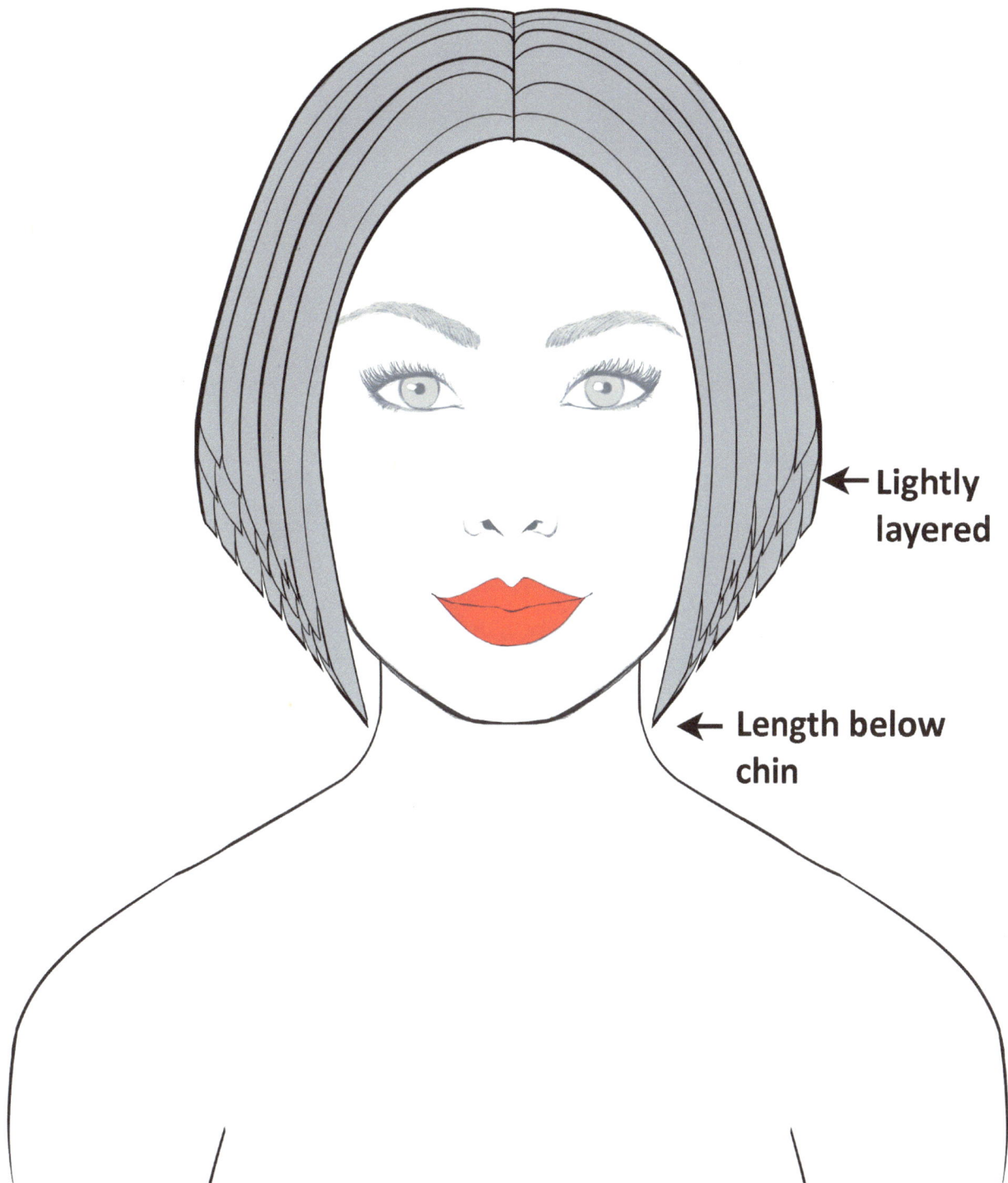

← **Lightly layered**

← **Length below chin**

SHORT LENGTH - CENTER PART

THE INVERTED BOB HAIRCUT

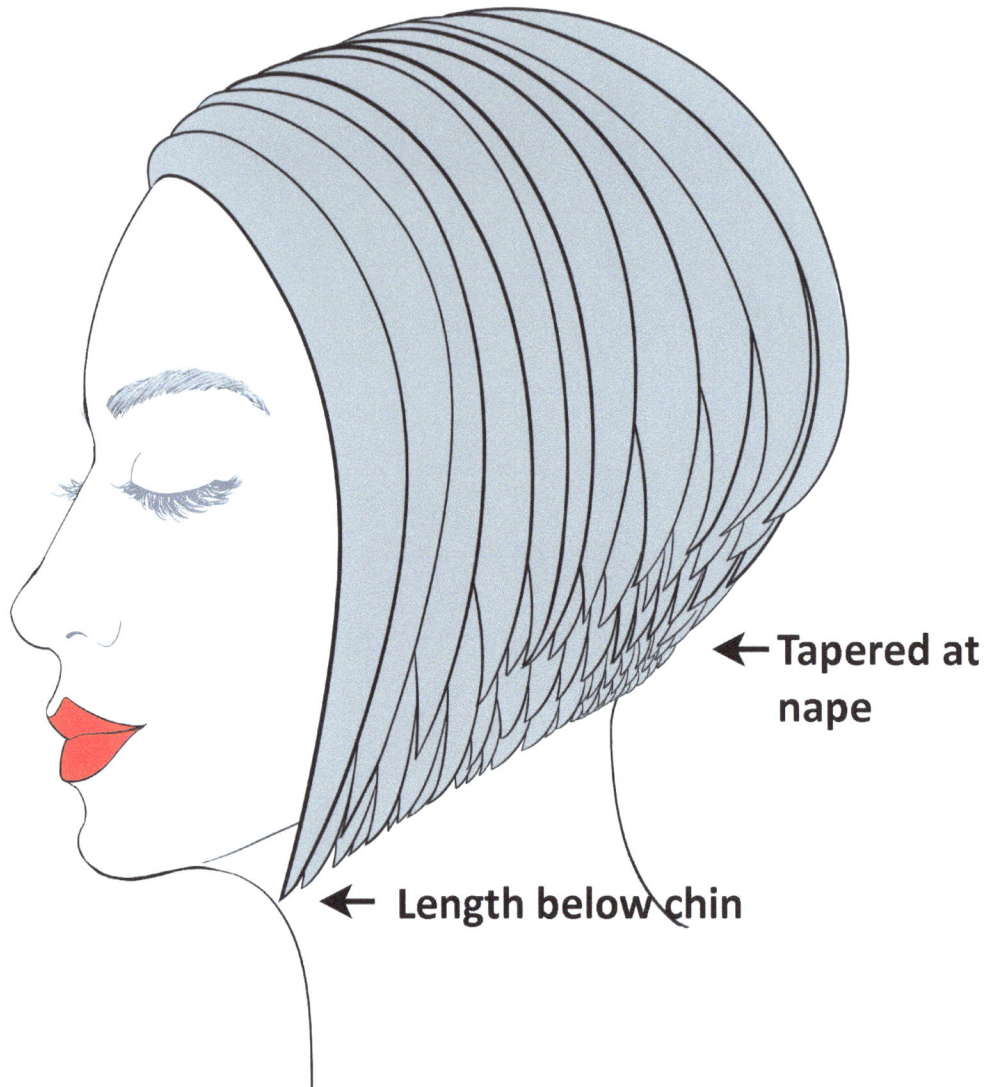

← Tapered at
nape

← Length below chin

SHORT LENGTH - CENTER PART

THE INVERTED BOB HAIRCUT

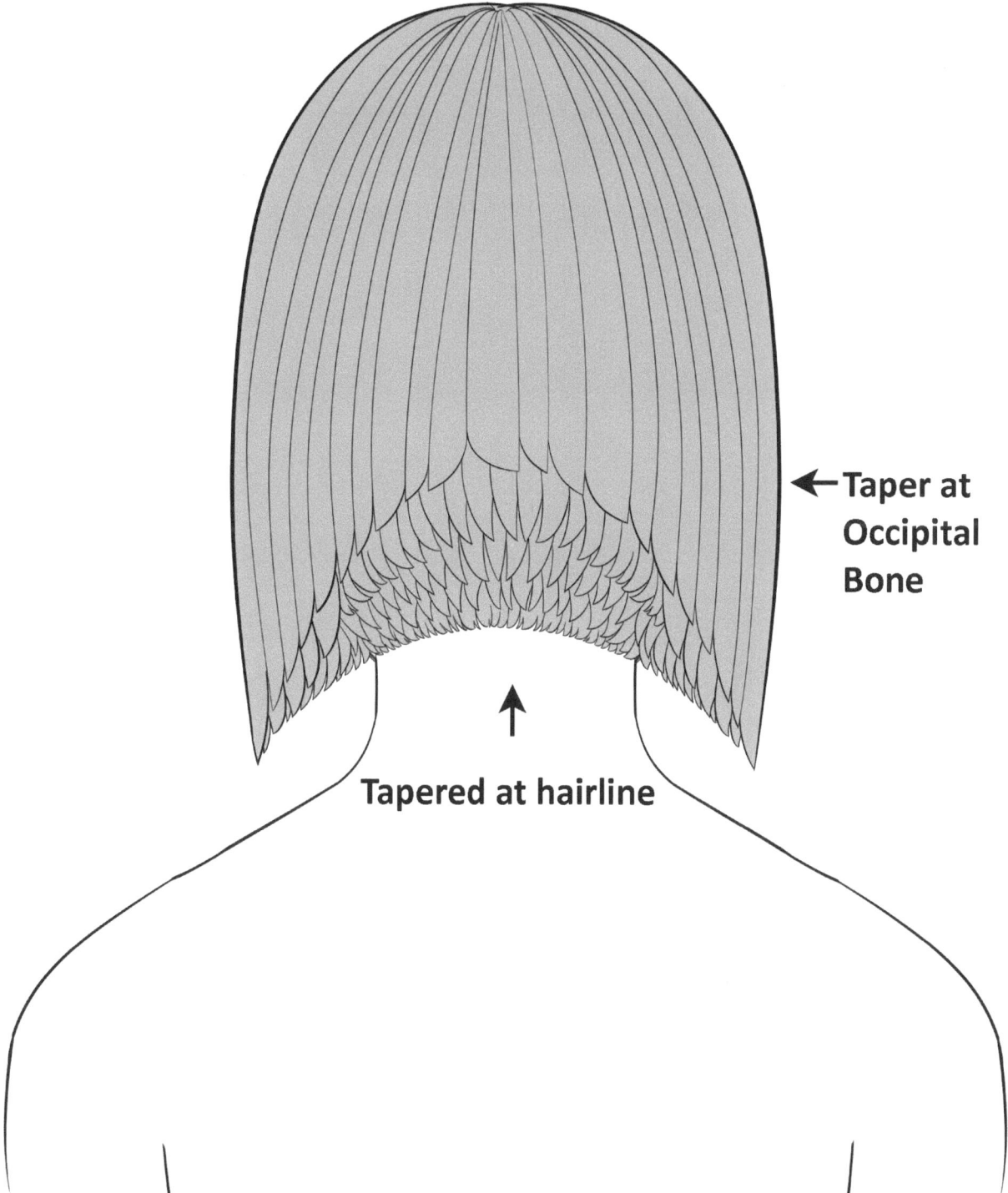

← Taper at Occipital Bone

↑ Tapered at hairline

SHORT LENGTH - CENTER PART

THE INVERTED BOB HAIRCUT

Disconnected Bang Options

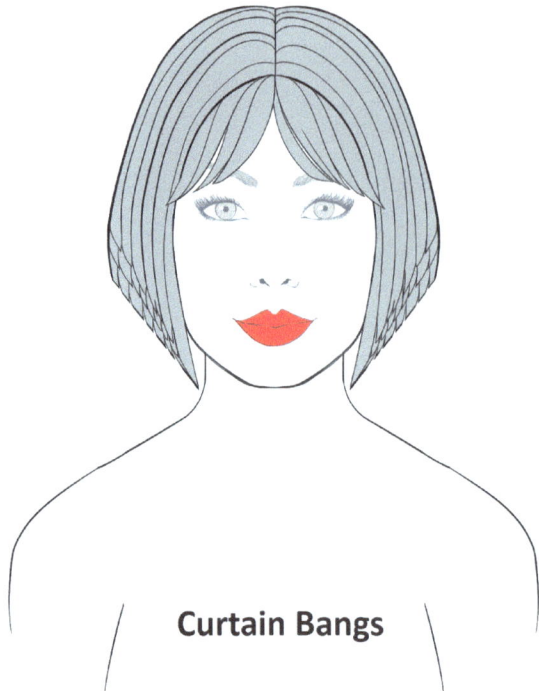

Curtain Bangs

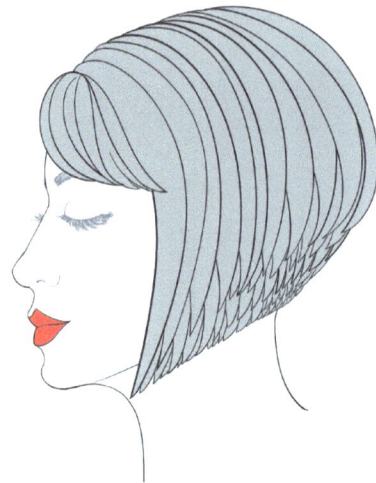

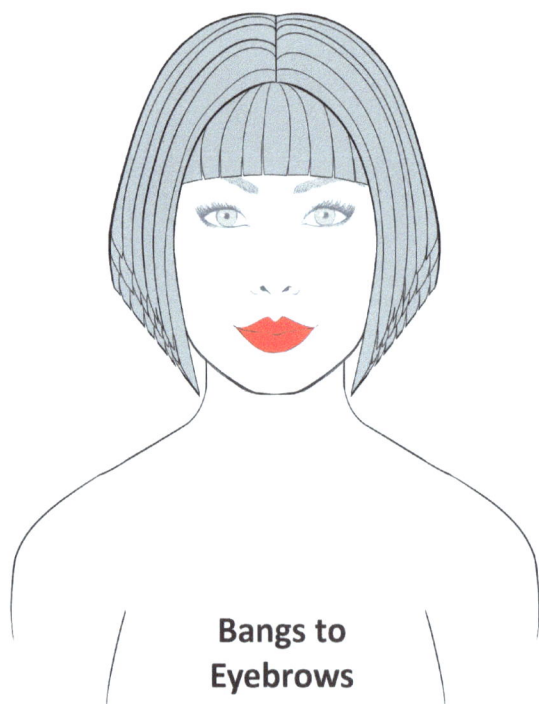

Curtain Bangs

Bangs to Eyebrows

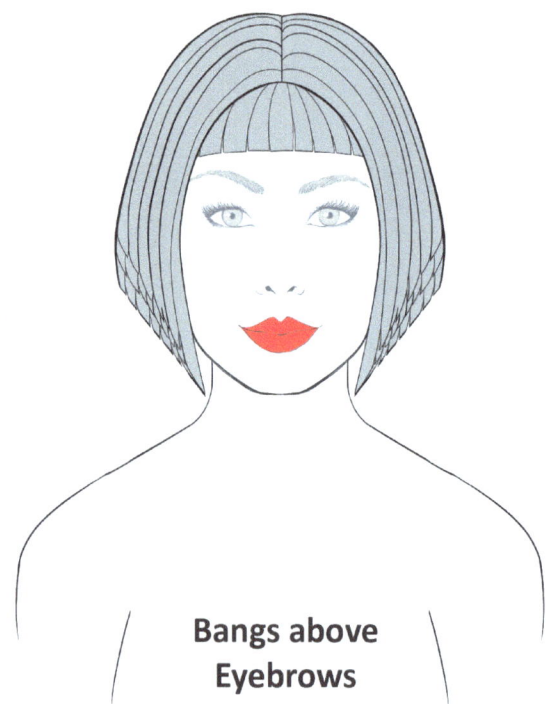

Bangs above Eyebrows

SHORT LENGTH - CENTER PART

THE INVERTED BOB HAIRCUT

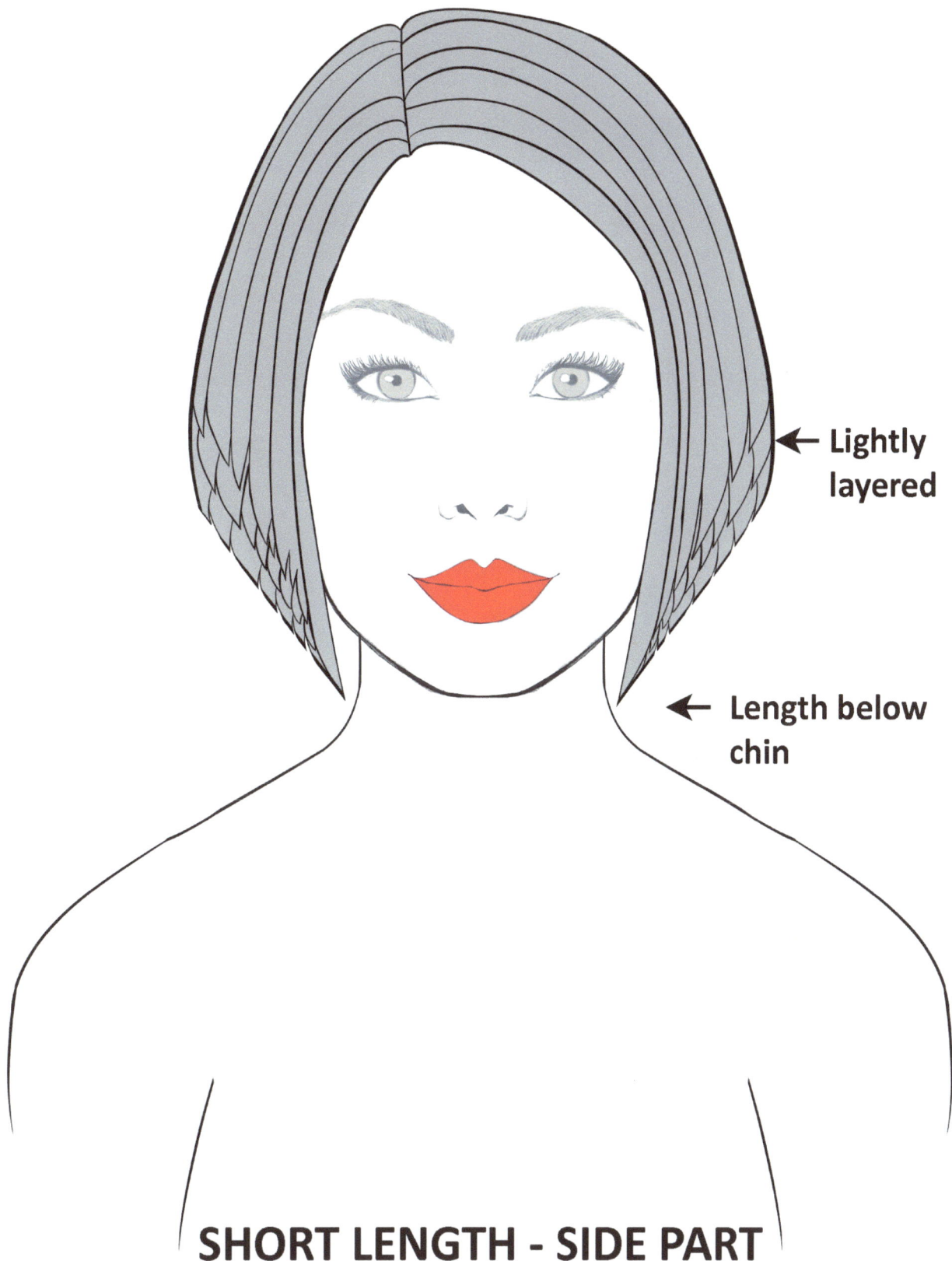

← **Lightly layered**

← **Length below chin**

SHORT LENGTH - SIDE PART

THE INVERTED BOB HAIRCUT

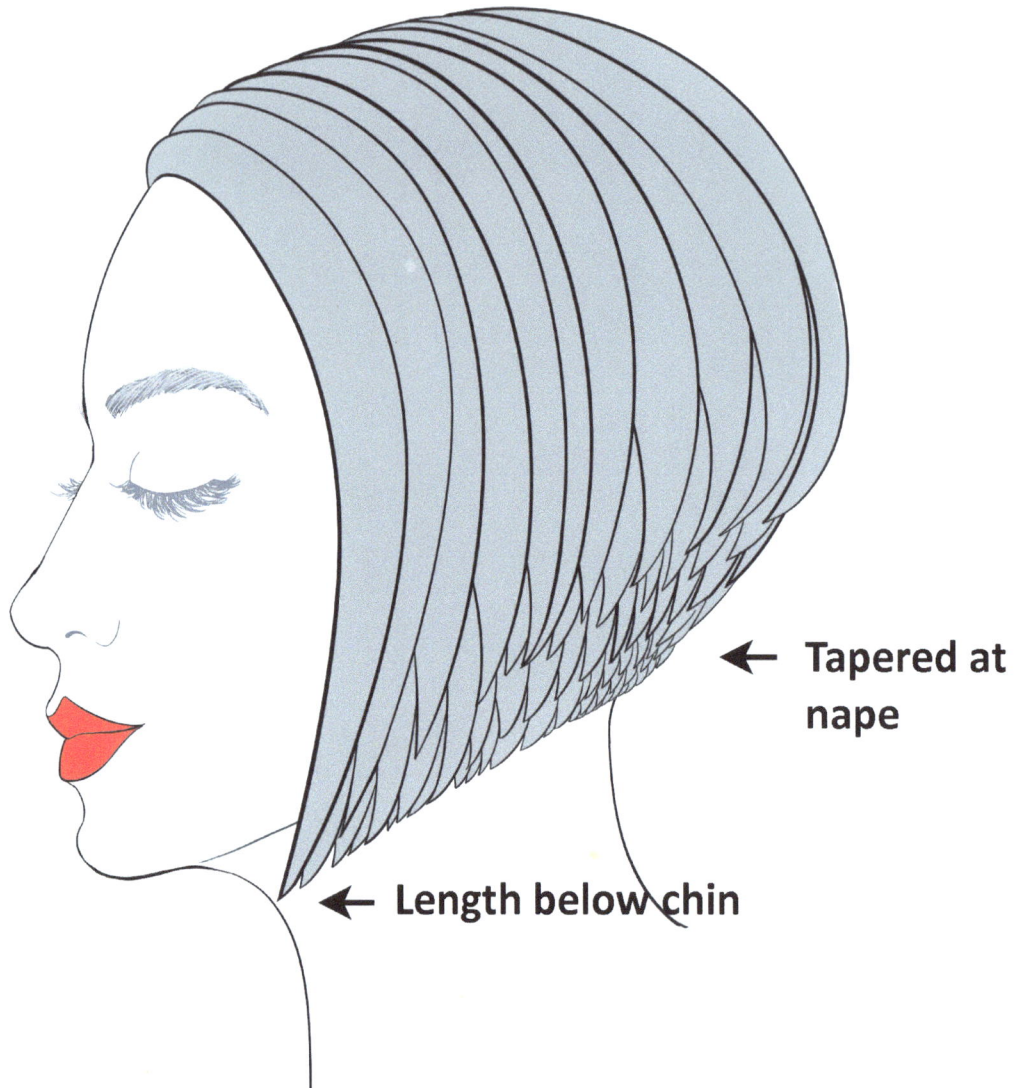

← Tapered at nape

← Length below chin

SHORT LENGTH - SIDE PART

THE INVERTED BOB HAIRCUT

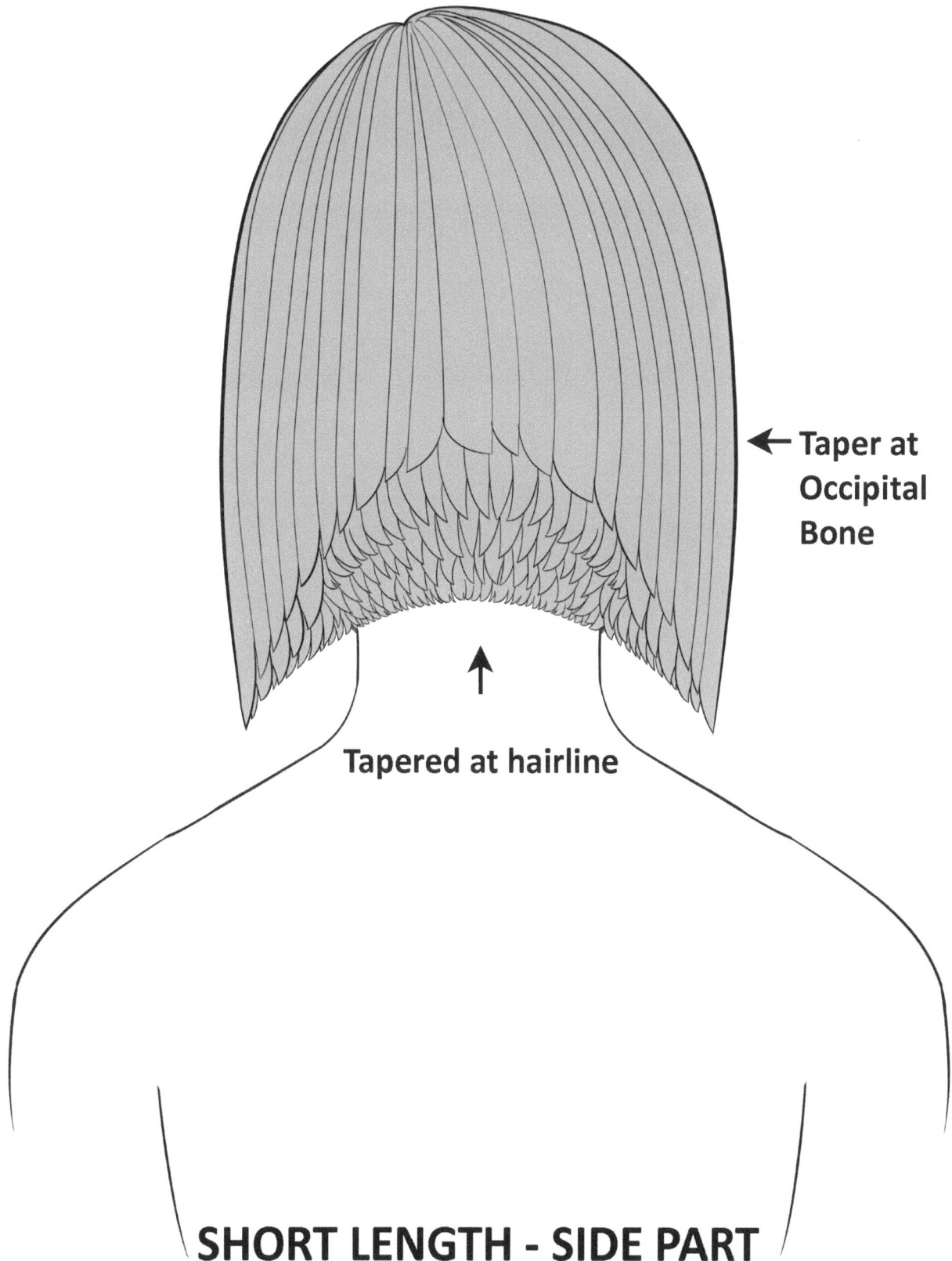

← Taper at Occipital Bone

Tapered at hairline

SHORT LENGTH - SIDE PART

THE INVERTED BOB HAIRCUT

Disconnected Bang Options

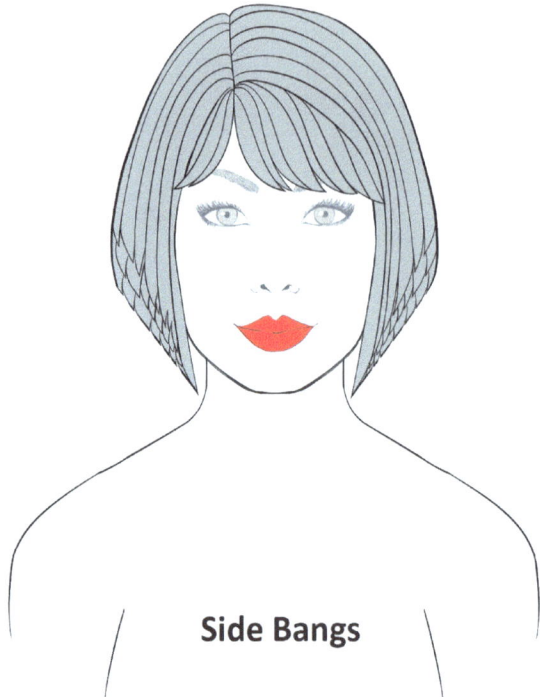

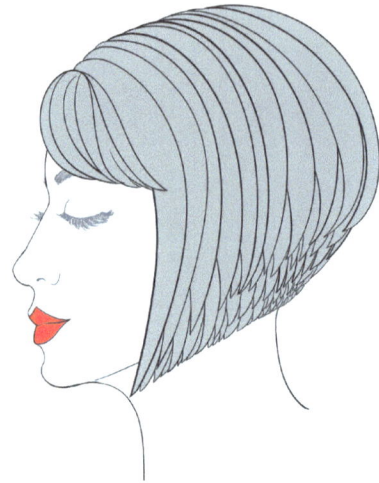

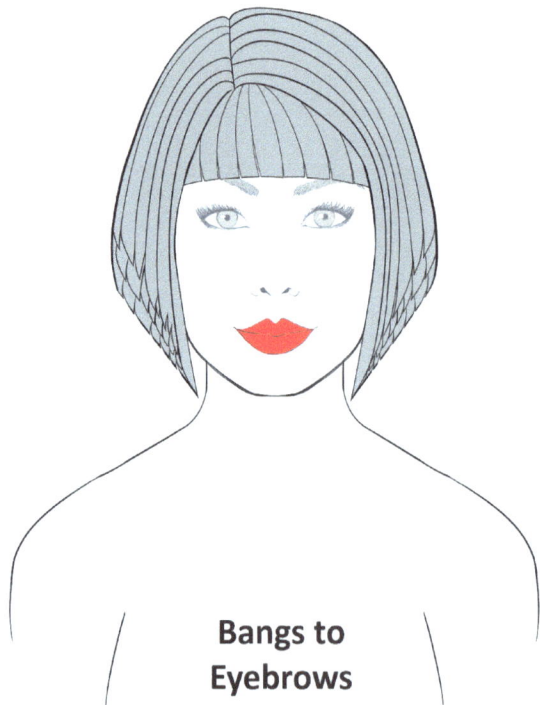

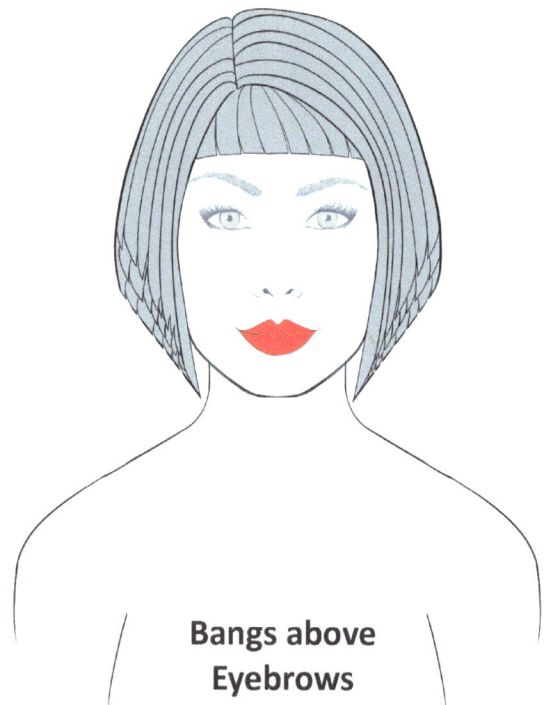

Side Bangs

Side Bangs

Bangs to Eyebrows

Bangs above Eyebrows

SHORT LENGTH - SIDE PART

THE INVERTED BOB HAIRCUT

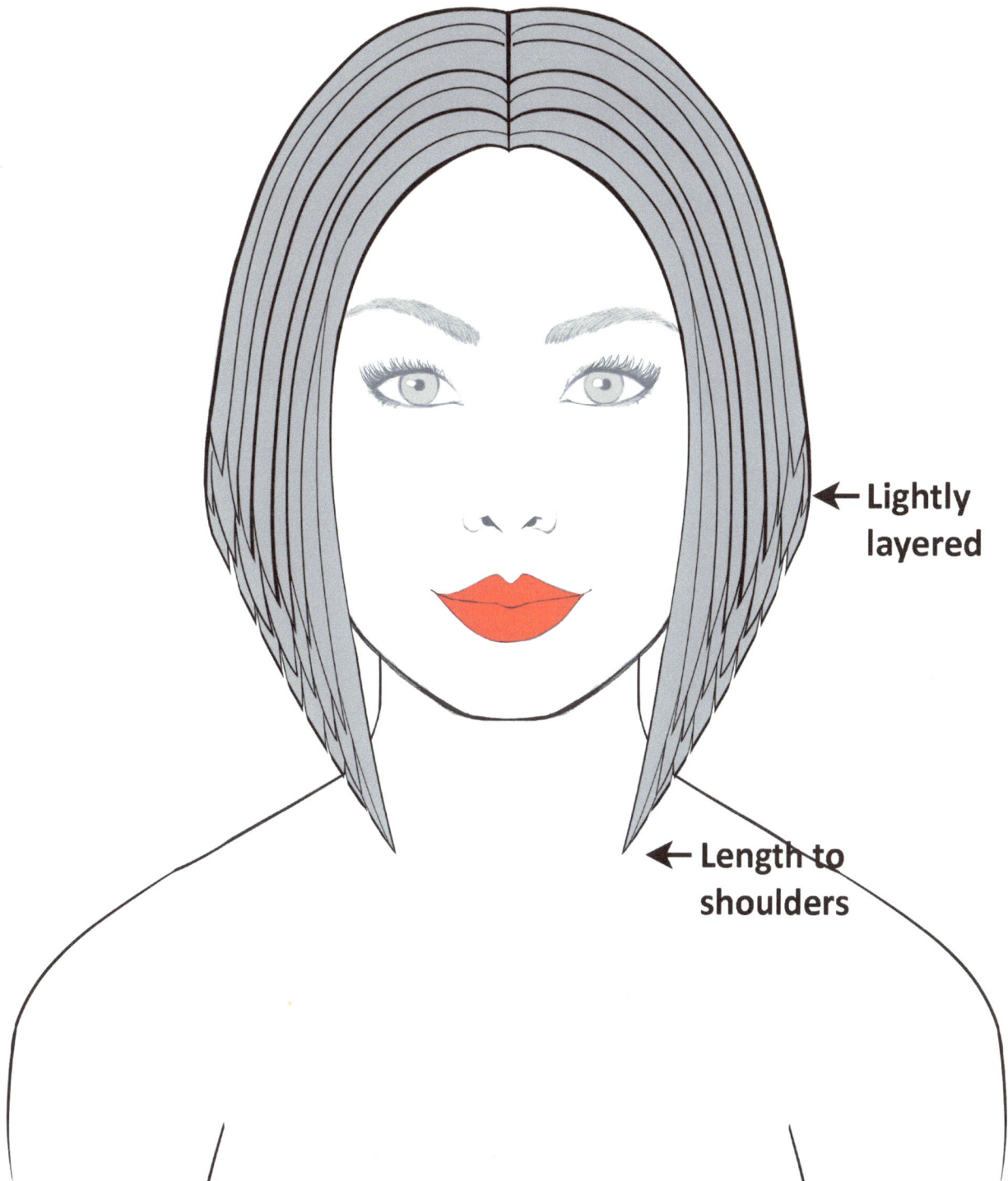

← Lightly layered

← Length to shoulders

MEDIUM LENGTH - CENTER PART

THE INVERTED BOB HAIRCUT

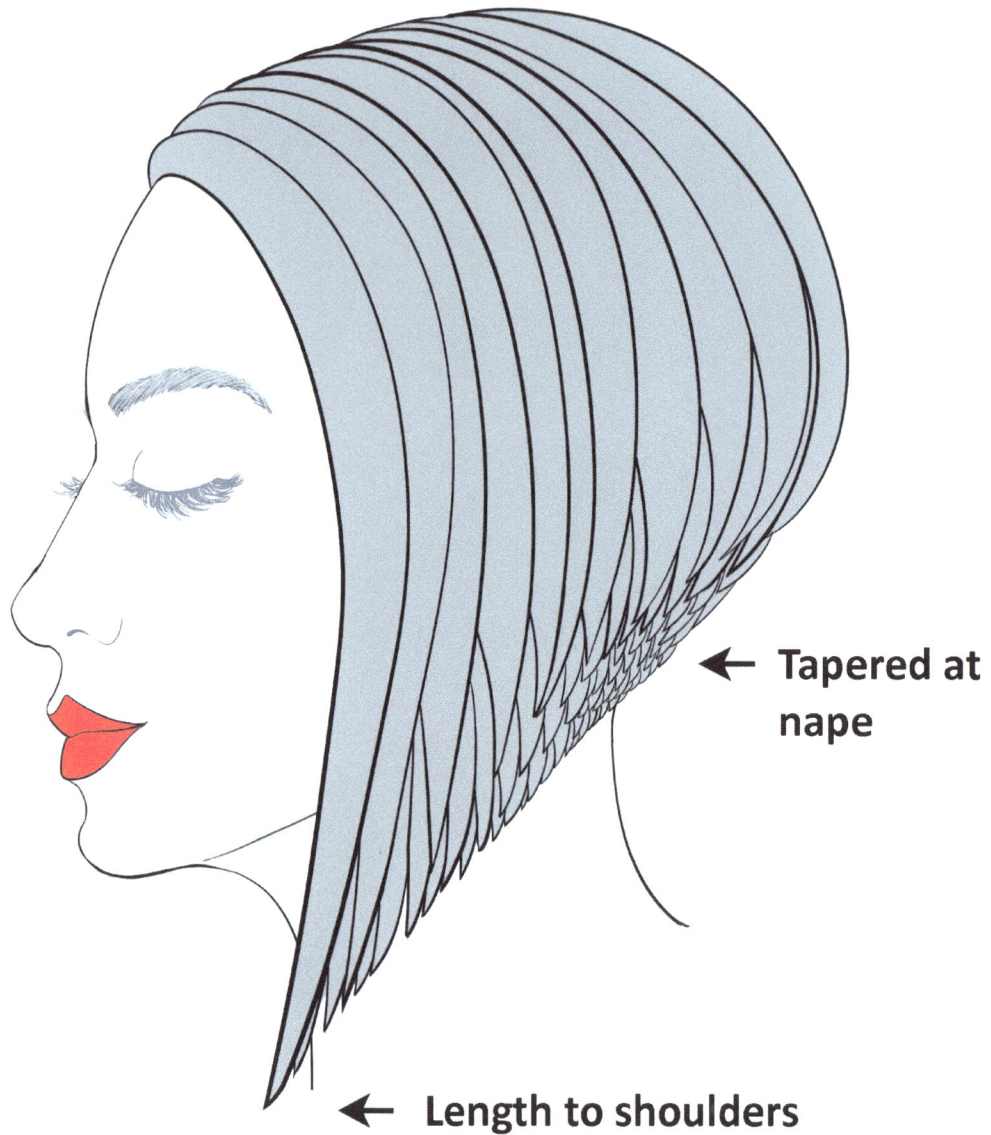

← **Tapered at nape**

← **Length to shoulders**

MEDIUM LENGTH - CENTER PART

THE INVERTED BOB HAIRCUT

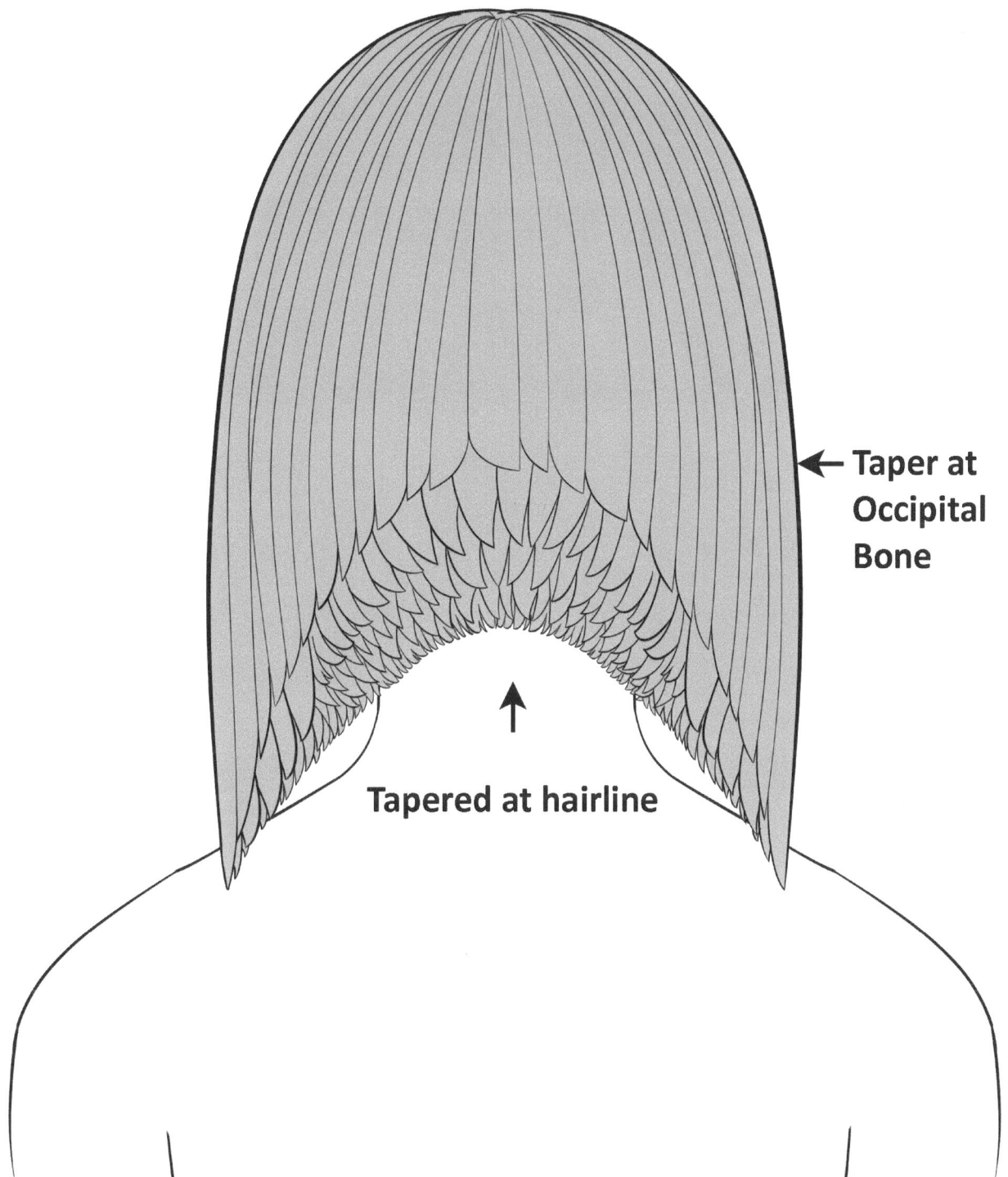

← Taper at
Occipital
Bone

↑

Tapered at hairline

MEDIUM LENGTH - CENTER PART

THE INVERTED BOB HAIRCUT

Disconnected Bang Options

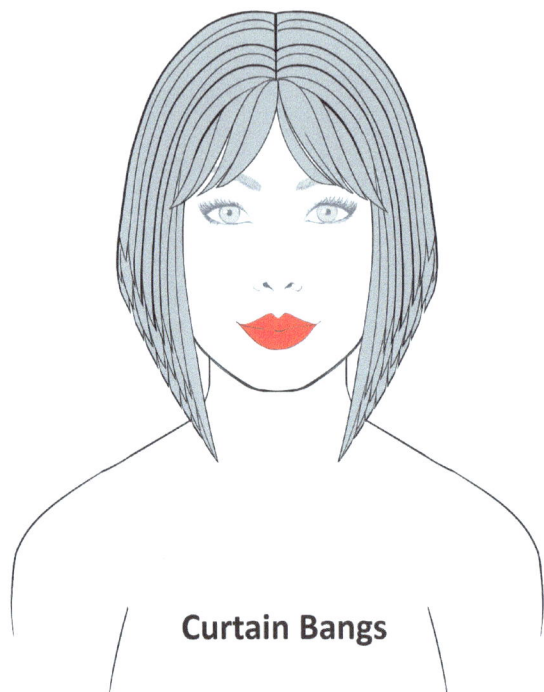

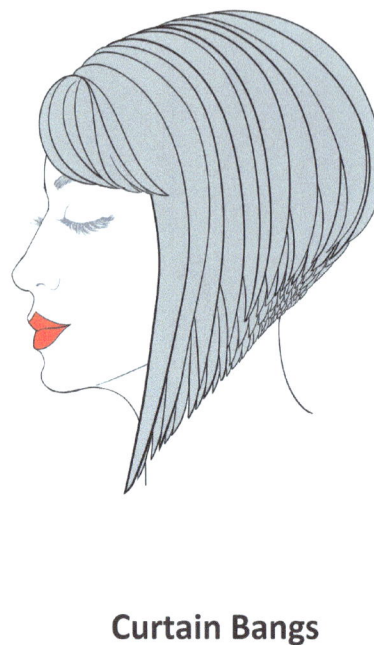

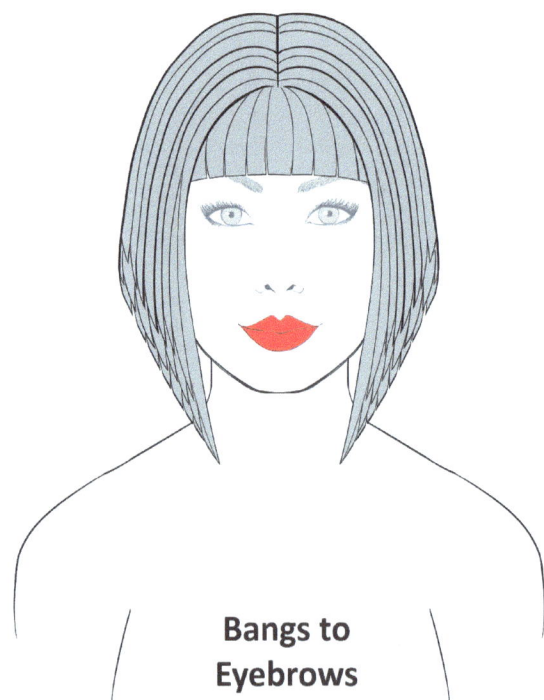

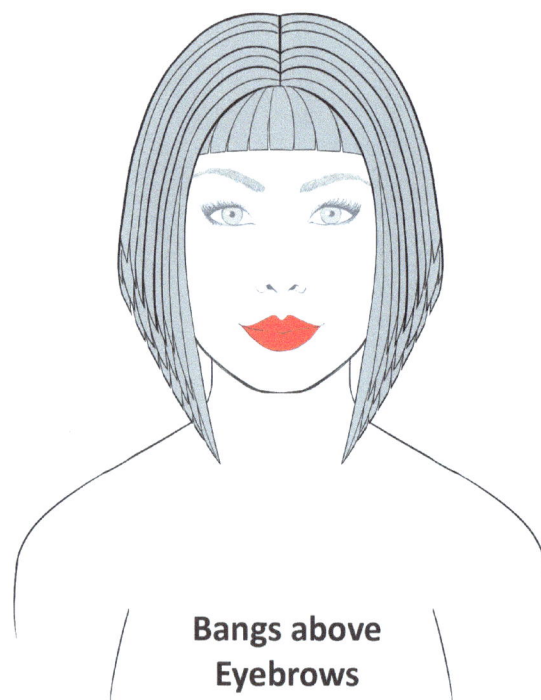

Curtain Bangs

Curtain Bangs

**Bangs to
Eyebrows**

**Bangs above
Eyebrows**

MEDIUM LENGTH - CENTER PART

THE INVERTED BOB HAIRCUT

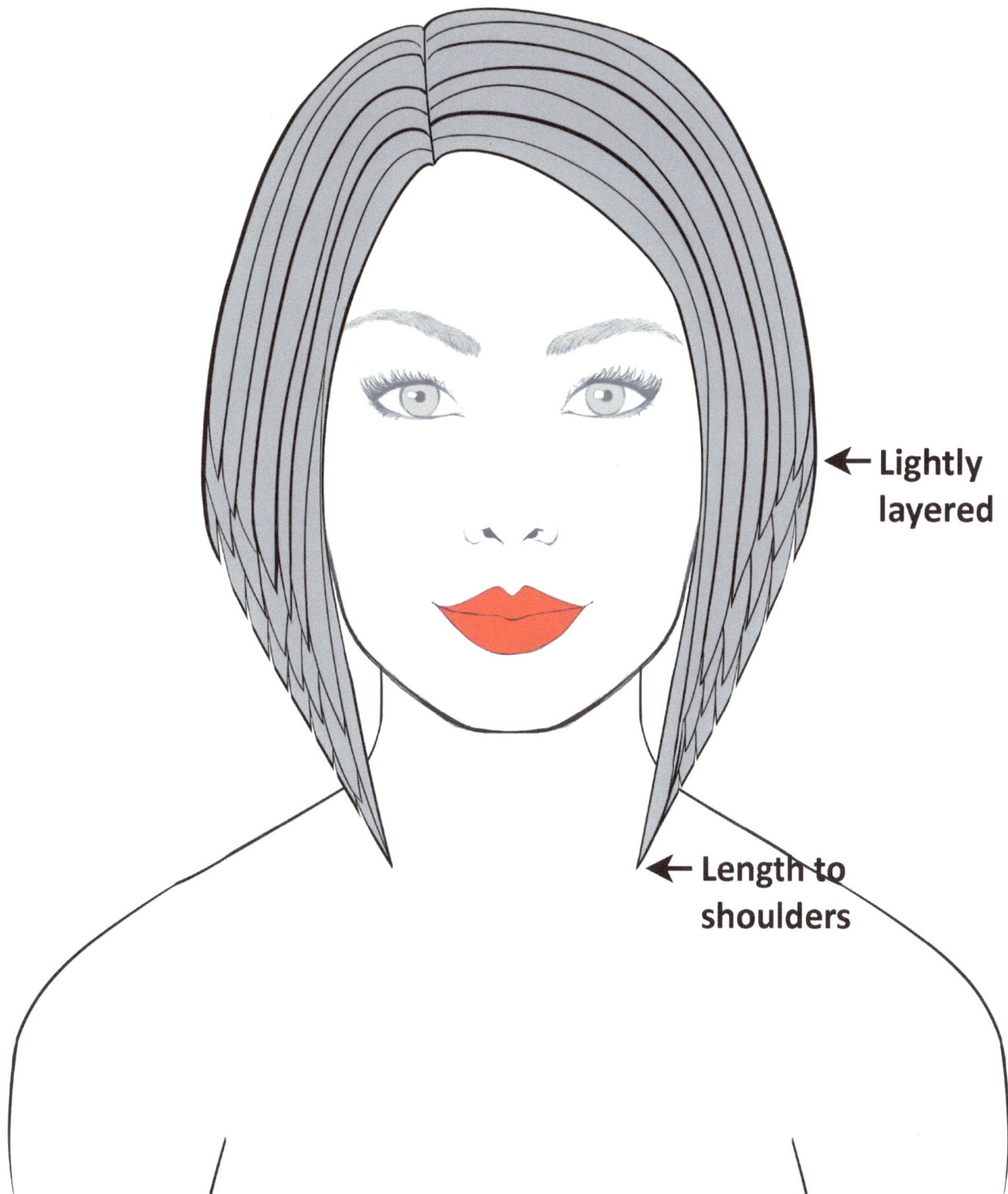

← Lightly layered

← Length to shoulders

MEDIUM LENGTH - SIDE PART

THE INVERTED BOB HAIRCUT

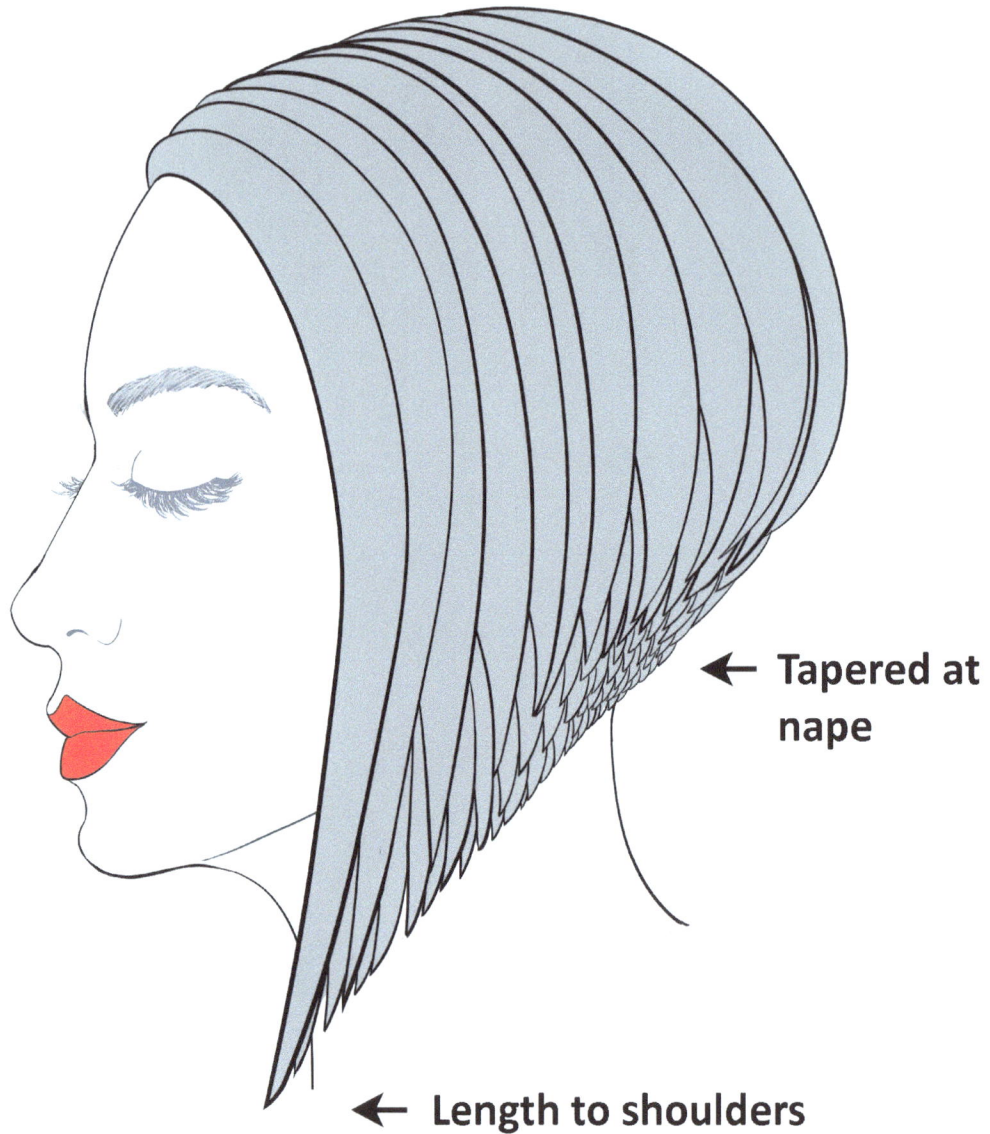

← Tapered at nape

← Length to shoulders

MEDIUM LENGTH - SIDE PART

THE INVERTED BOB HAIRCUT

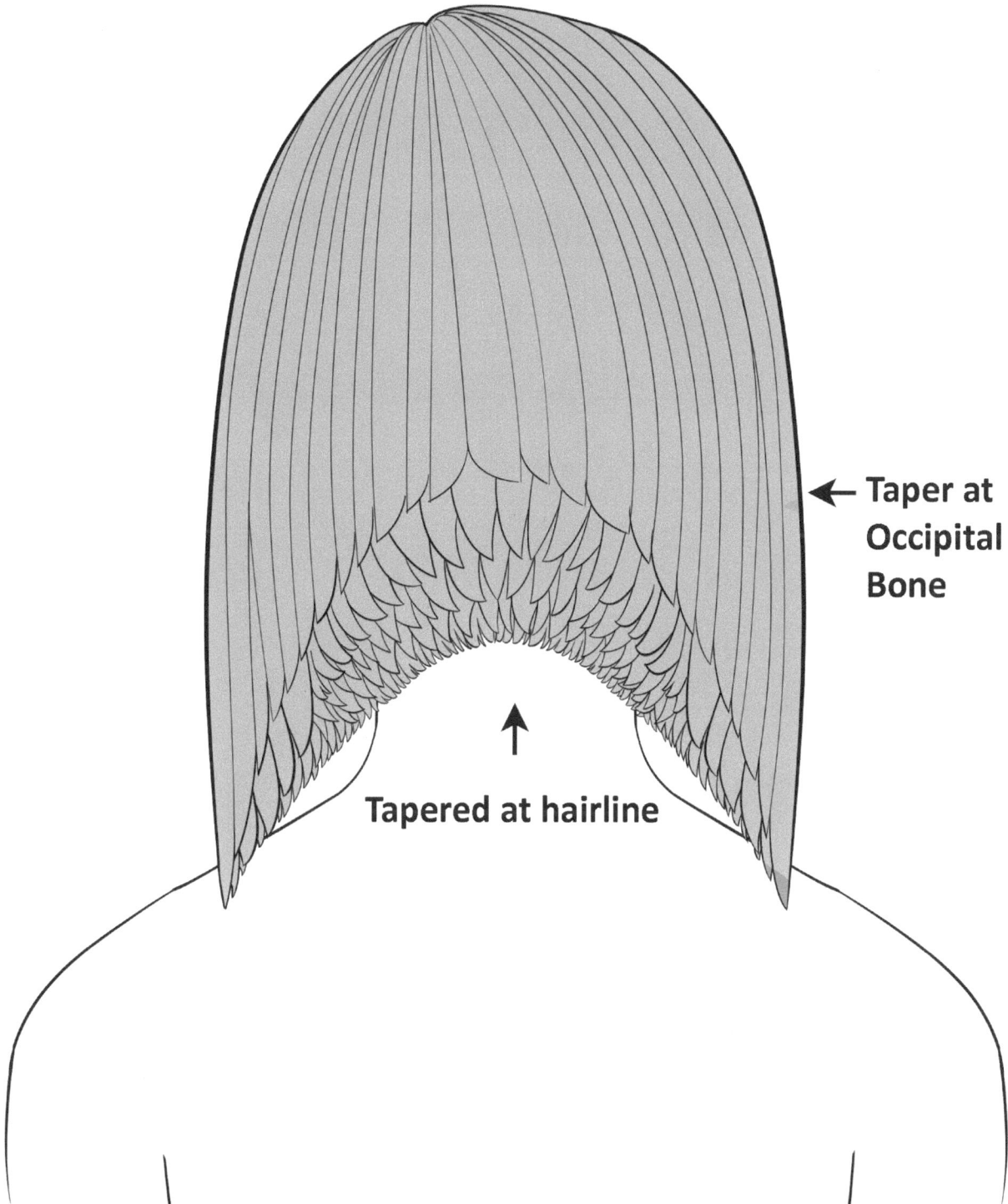

← Taper at
Occipital
Bone

↑
Tapered at hairline

MEDIUM LENGTH - SIDE PART

THE INVERTED BOB HAIRCUT

Disconnected Bang Options

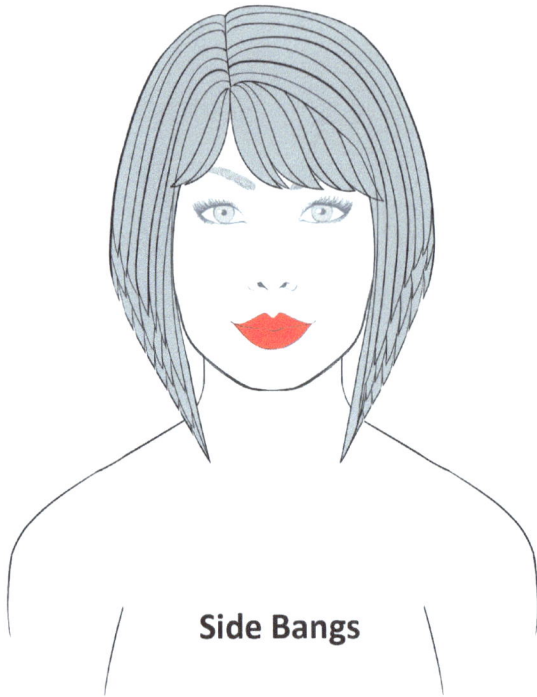

Side Bangs

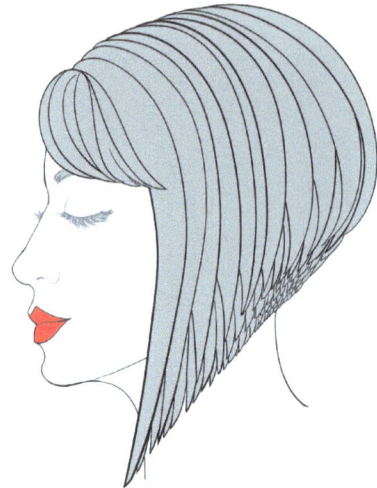

Side Bangs

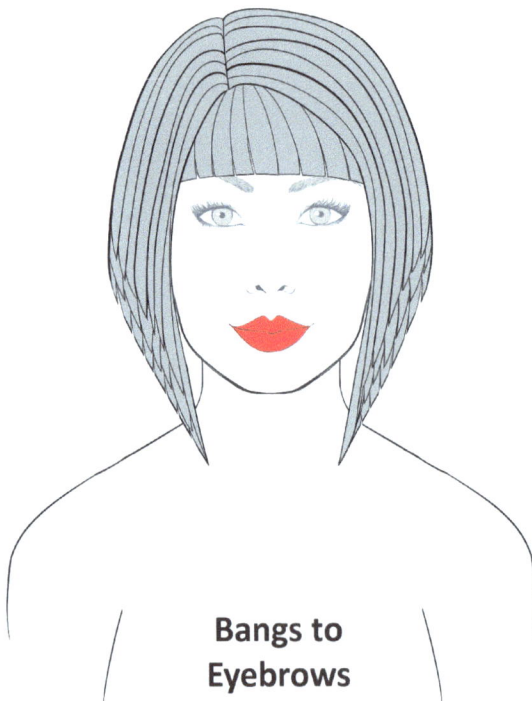

Bangs to Eyebrows

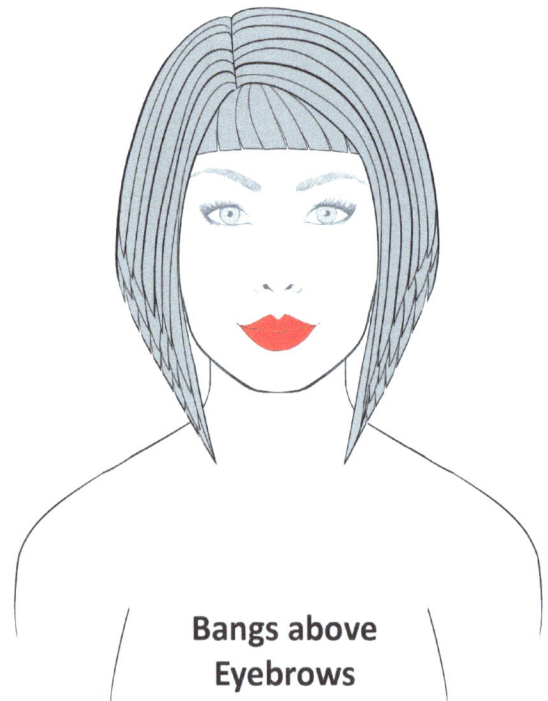

Bangs above Eyebrows

MEDIUM LENGTH - SIDE PART

Chapter 6
THE BI-LEVEL HAIRCUT

This elegant haircut offers a polished finish with little effort.
And, it's great for showing off your earrings!

- **LENGTH-** The Bi-Level Haircut looks great in short lengths and medium lengths.

- **PART-** This haircut has a changeable part.

- **BANGS-** The bangs can be shorter or longer to suit your personal preference.

- **LAYERS-** Choose short layers or long layers to serve your unique hair texture and hair type.

- **EARS-** Choose hair above the ear, top of the ear covered, half of the ear covered, or all of the ear covered.

- **STYLING-** The Bi-Level Haircut is a snap to style. A fast blow dry and if needed use a curling iron or flat iron for a polished finish.

THE BI-LEVEL HAIRCUT

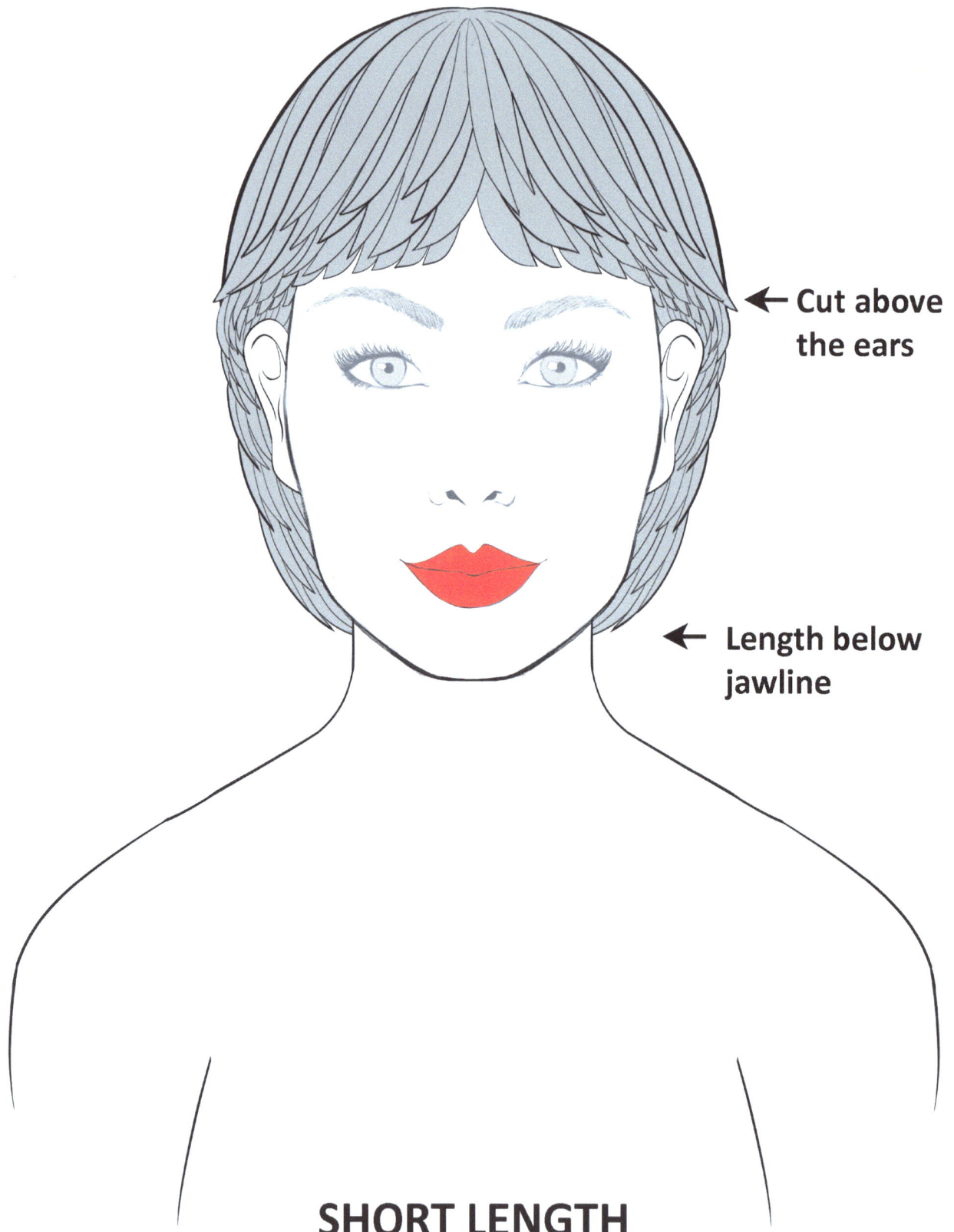

← Cut above
the ears

← Length below
jawline

SHORT LENGTH

THE BI-LEVEL HAIRCUT

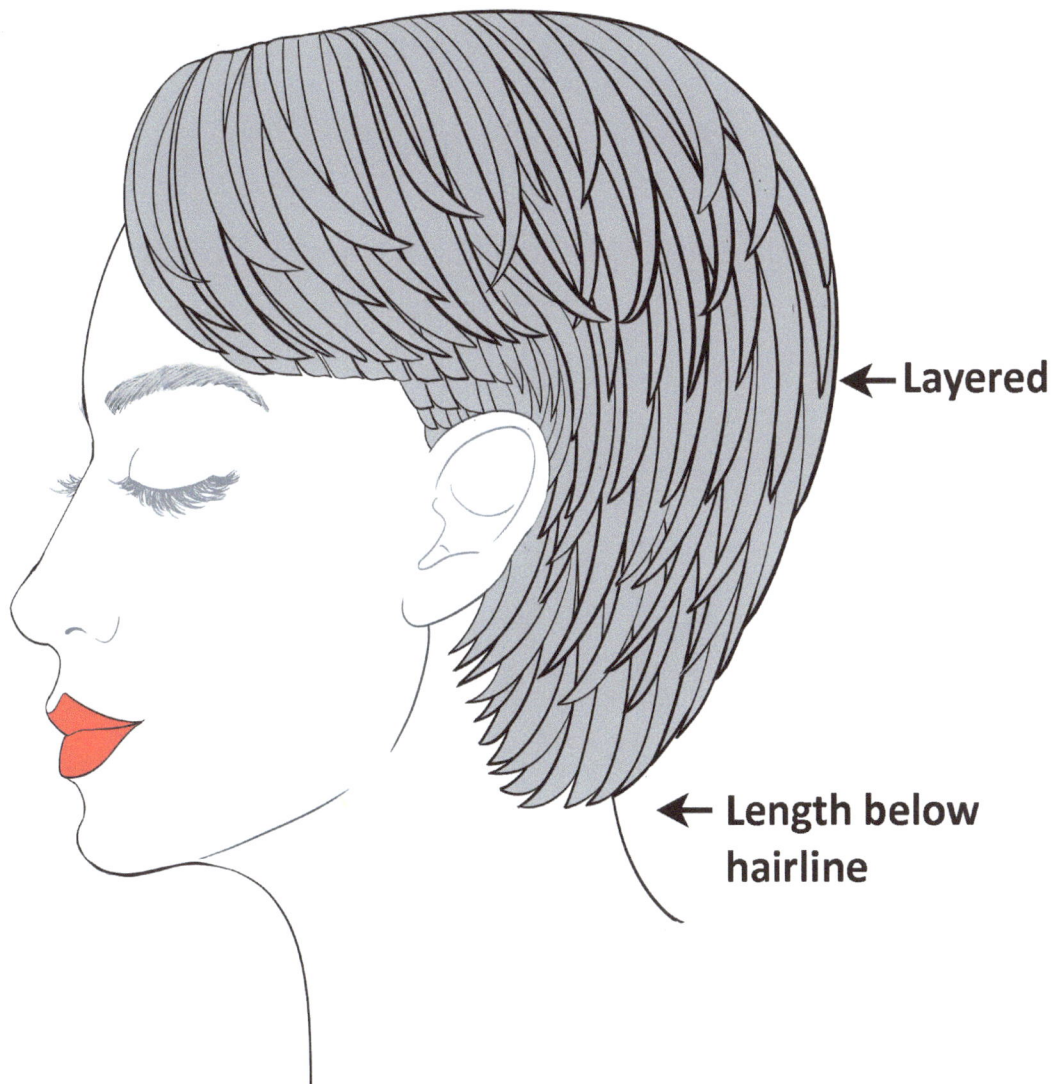

← Layered

← Length below
hairline

SHORT LENGTH

THE BI-LEVEL HAIRCUT

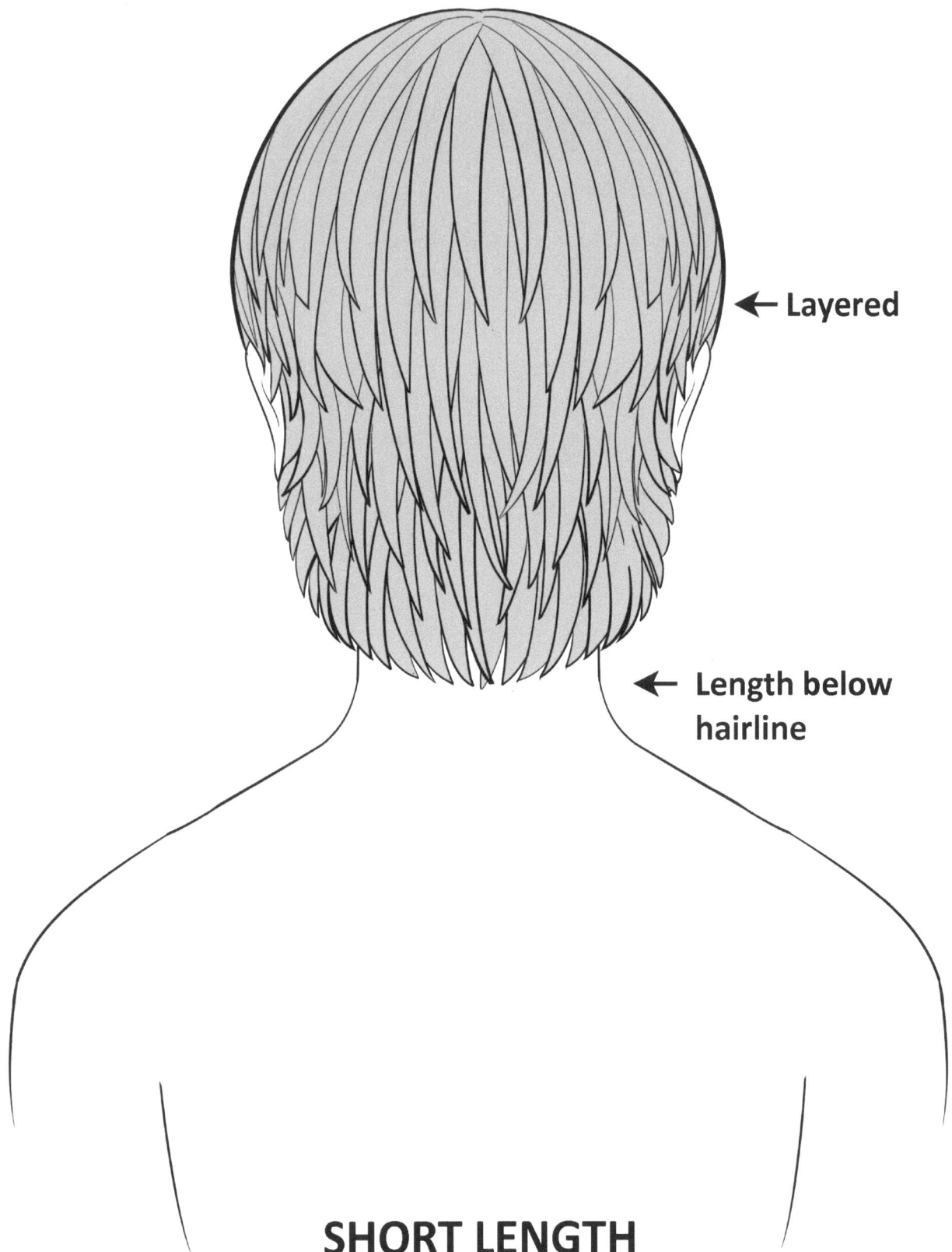

← Layered

← Length below
hairline

SHORT LENGTH

THE BI-LEVEL HAIRCUT

Ear Options

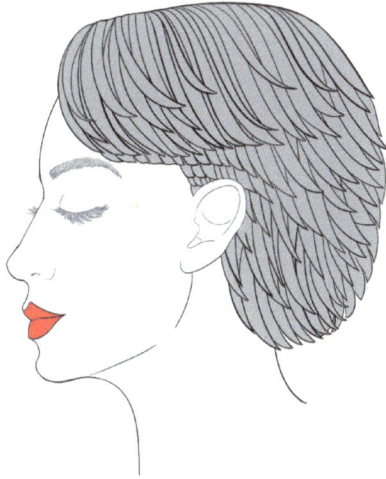

Above the Ear

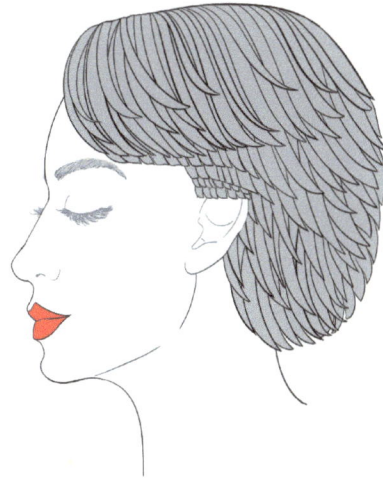

Top of Ear Covered

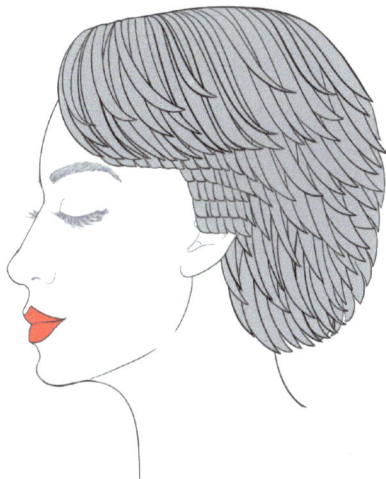

Half of Ear Covered

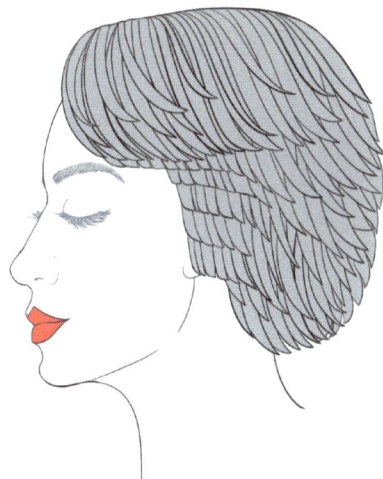

Whole Ear Covered

SHORT LENGTH

THE BI-LEVEL HAIRCUT

Styling Options

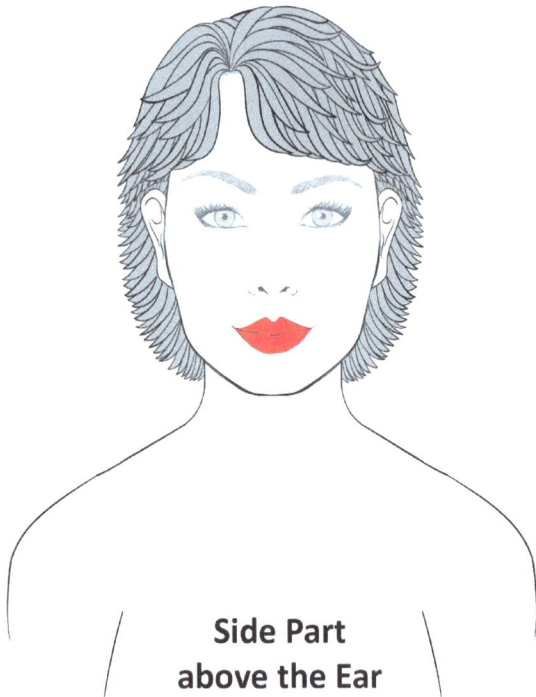

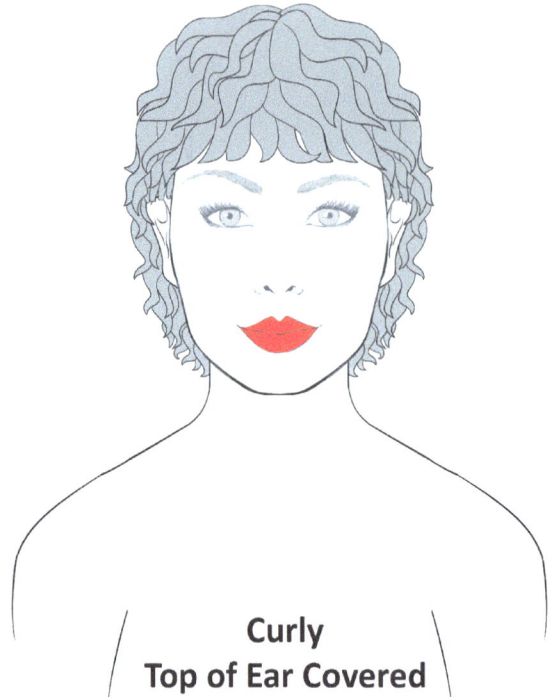

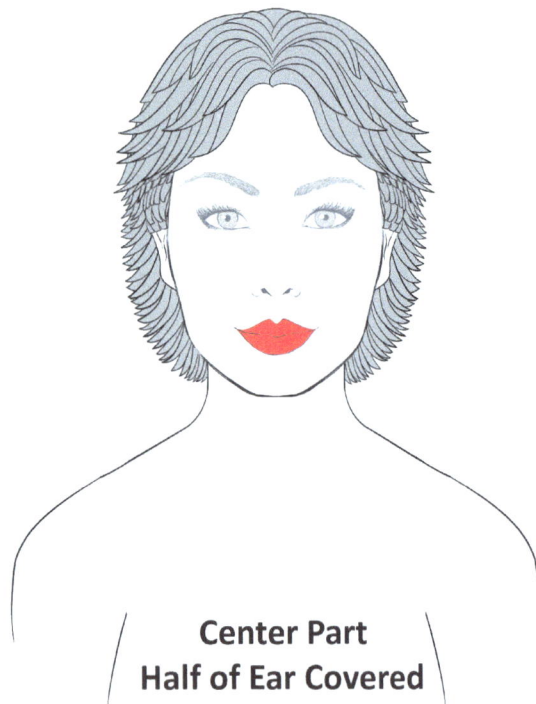

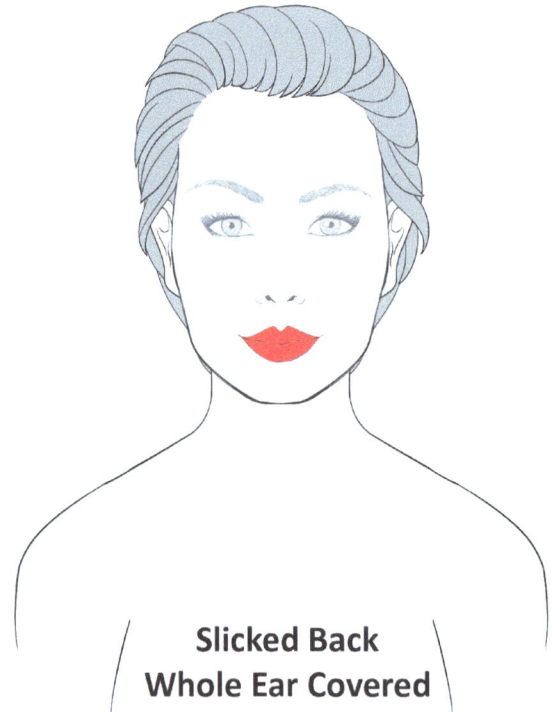

**Side Part
above the Ear**

**Curly
Top of Ear Covered**

**Center Part
Half of Ear Covered**

**Slicked Back
Whole Ear Covered**

SHORT LENGTH

THE BI-LEVEL HAIRCUT

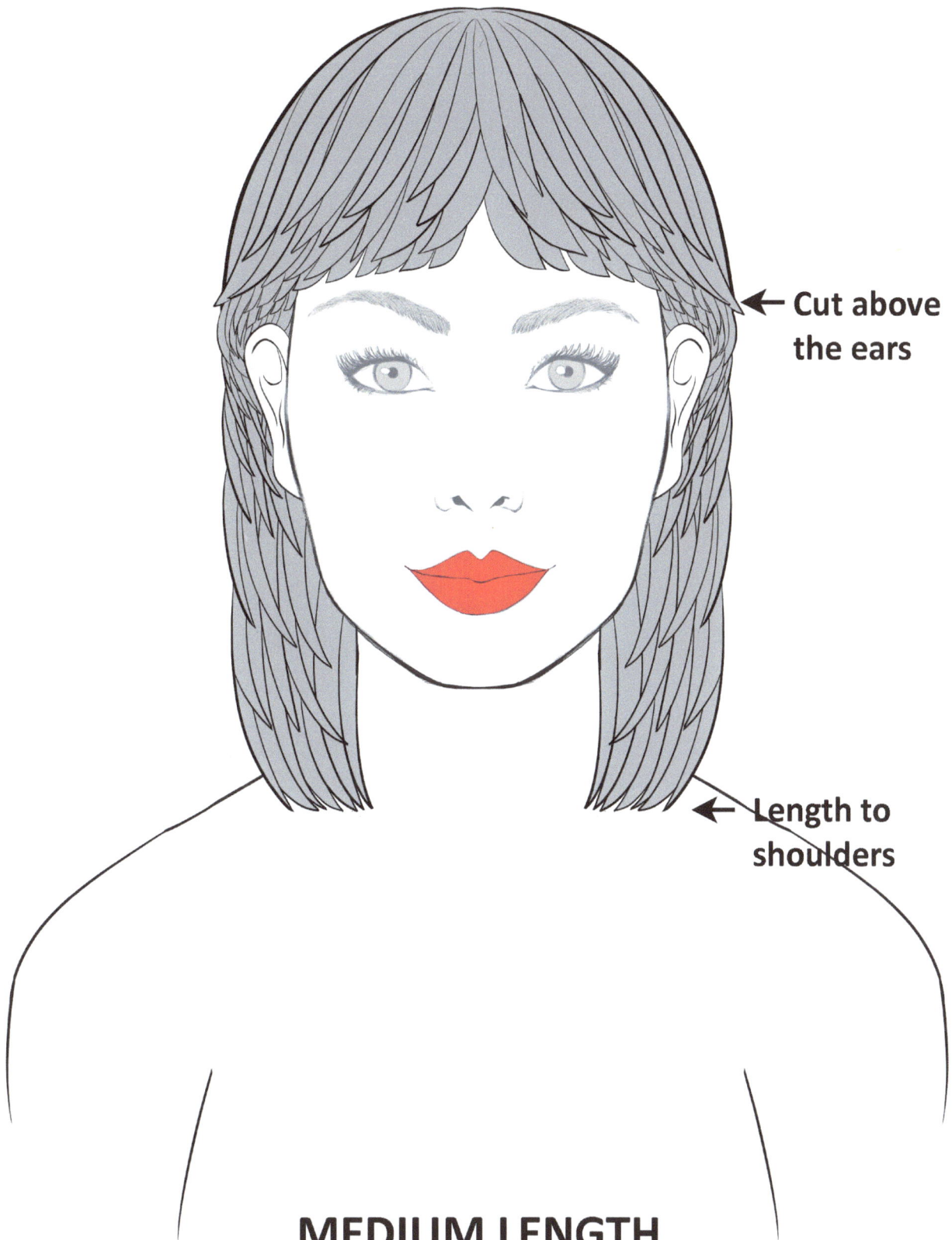

← Cut above
the ears

← Length to
shoulders

MEDIUM LENGTH

THE BI-LEVEL HAIRCUT

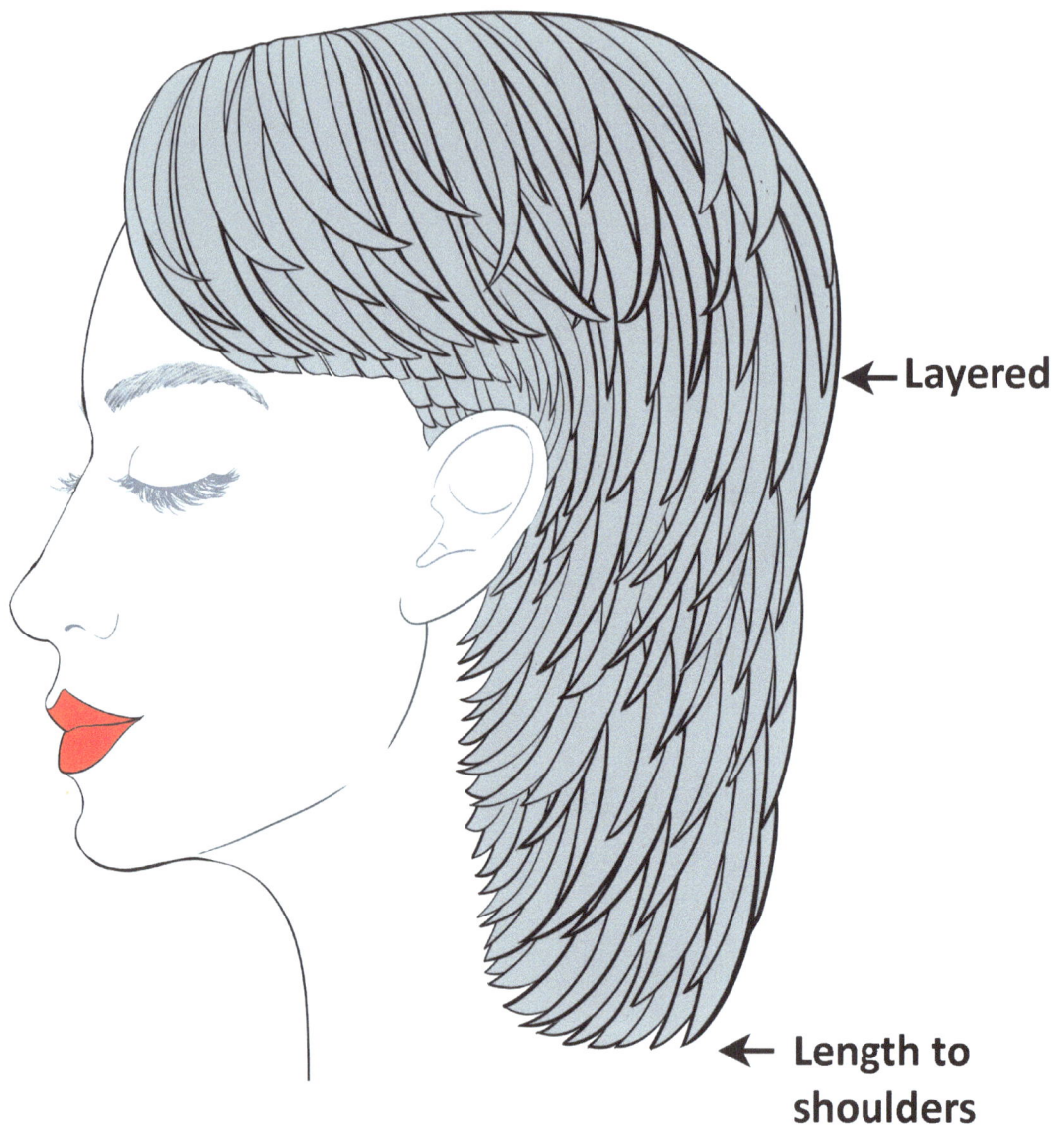

← Layered

← Length to shoulders

MEDIUM LENGTH

THE BI-LEVEL HAIRCUT

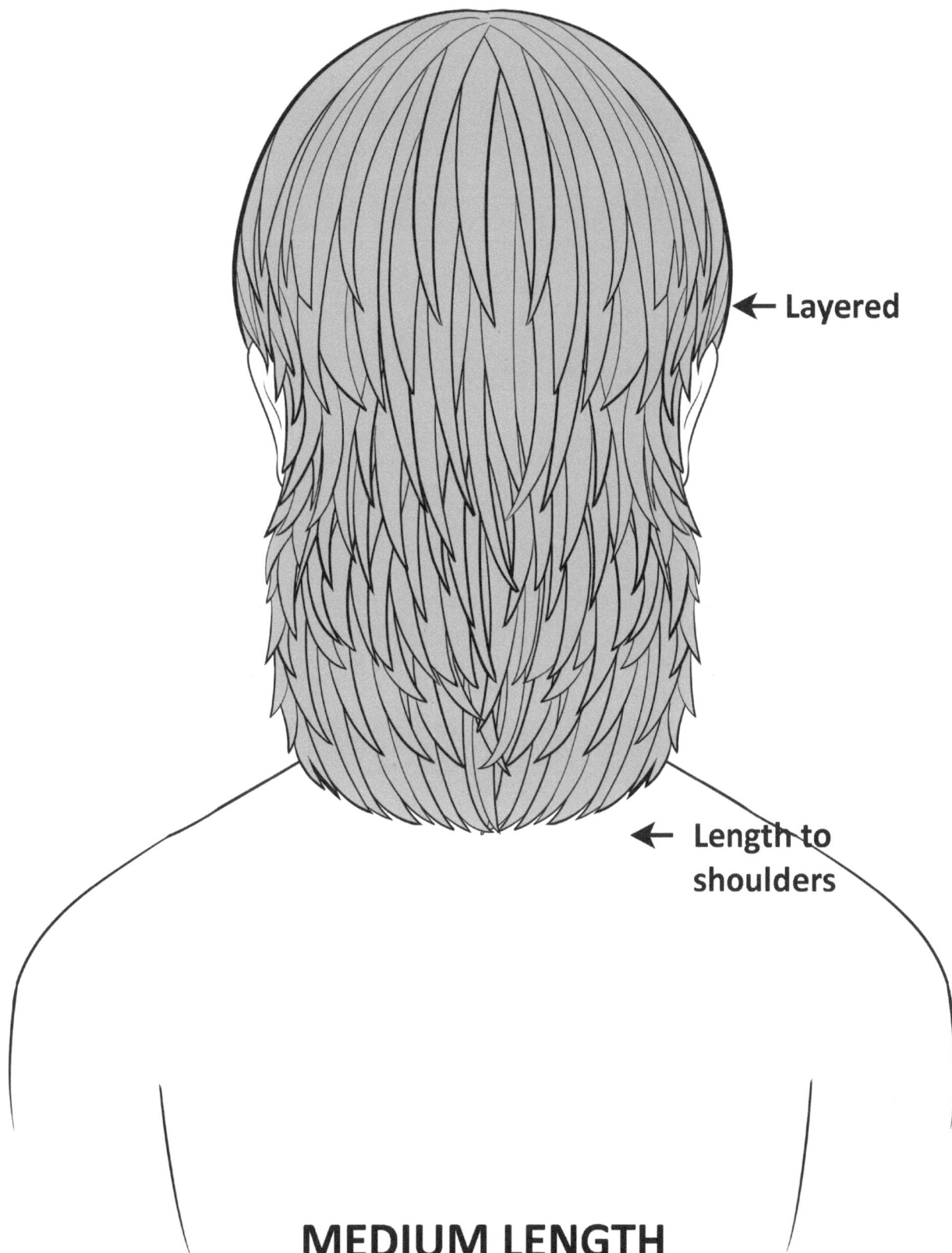

← Layered

← Length to shoulders

MEDIUM LENGTH

THE BI-LEVEL HAIRCUT

Ear Options

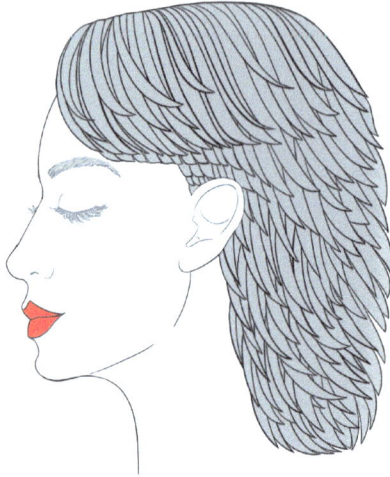

Above the Ear

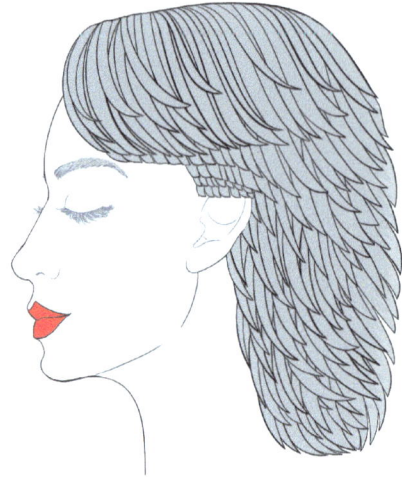

Top of Ear Covered

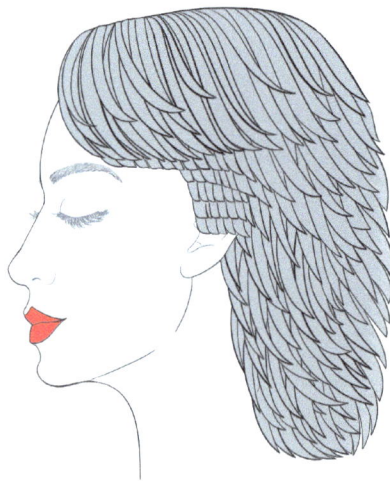

Half of Ear Covered

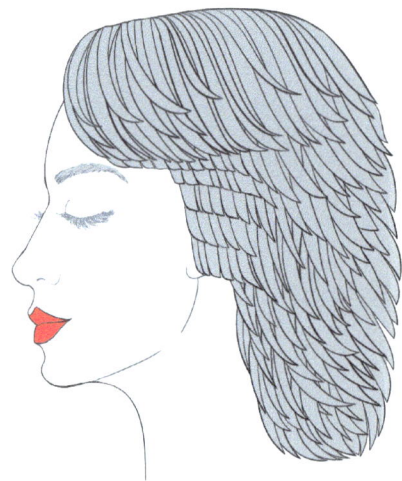

Whole Ear Covered

MEDIUM LENGTH

THE BI-LEVEL HAIRCUT

Styling Options

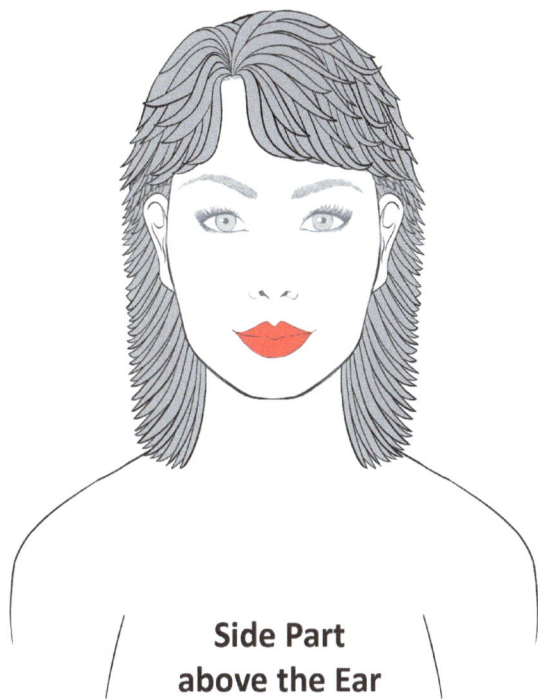

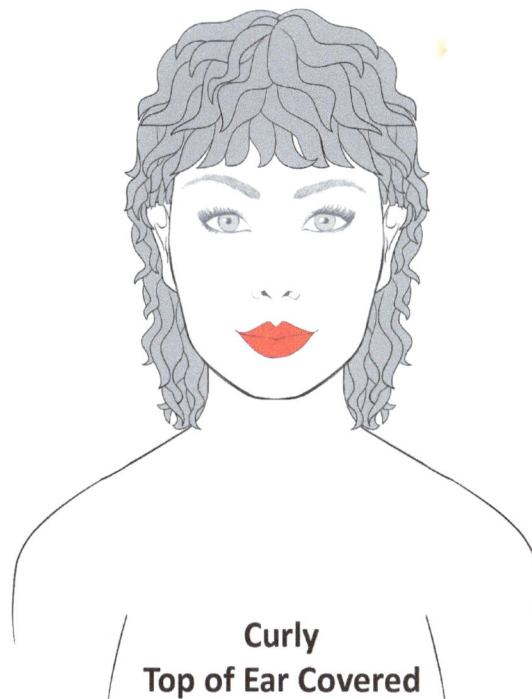

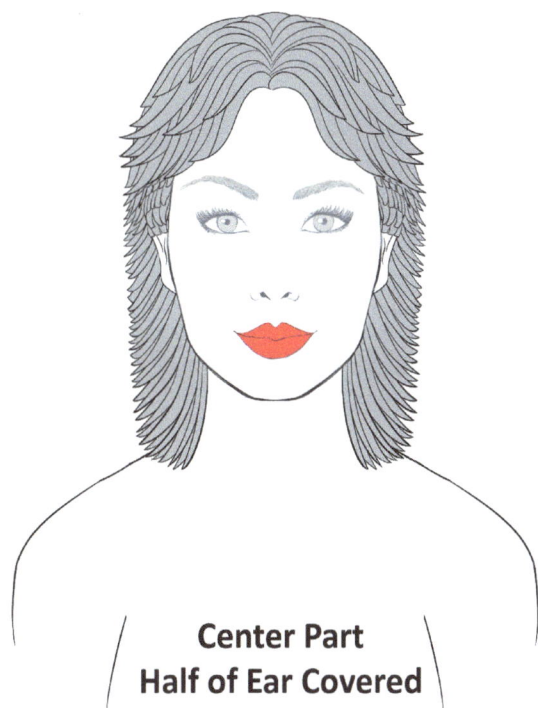

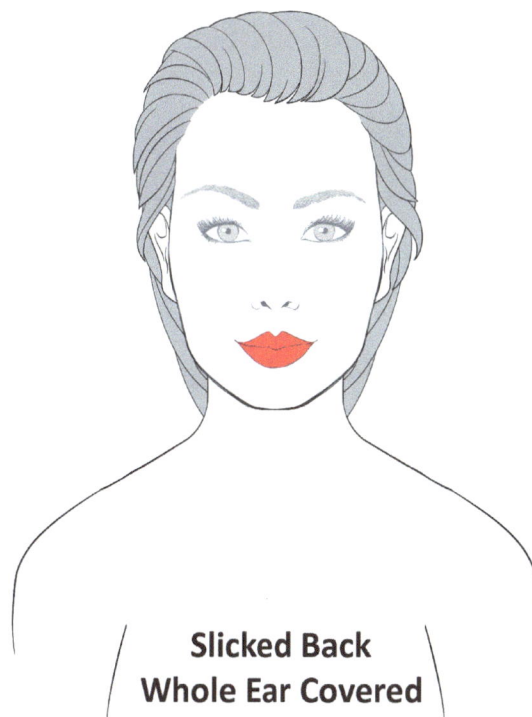

**Side Part
above the Ear**

**Curly
Top of Ear Covered**

**Center Part
Half of Ear Covered**

**Slicked Back
Whole Ear Covered**

MEDIUM LENGTH

Chapter 7
THE PIXIE HAIRCUT

This chic and sassy haircut offers lots of attitude. If you love your hair short, this is the haircut for you.

- **LENGTH-** The Pixie Haircut looks great in short lengths and medium lengths.

- **PART-** This haircut has a changeable part.

- **BANGS-** The bangs can be shorter or longer to suit your personal preference.

- **LAYERS-** Choose short layers or long layers to serve your unique hair texture and hair type.

- **EARS-** Choose pointed sideburns, angled sideburns, wispy sideburns, or top of the ear covered.

- **NAPE-** Choose tapered nape, square nape, round nape, or fringe nape.

- **STYLING-** The Pixie Haircut has a super quick styling time. A quick blow dry and maybe a little fine tuning with a flat iron or a curling iron.

THE PIXIE HAIRCUT

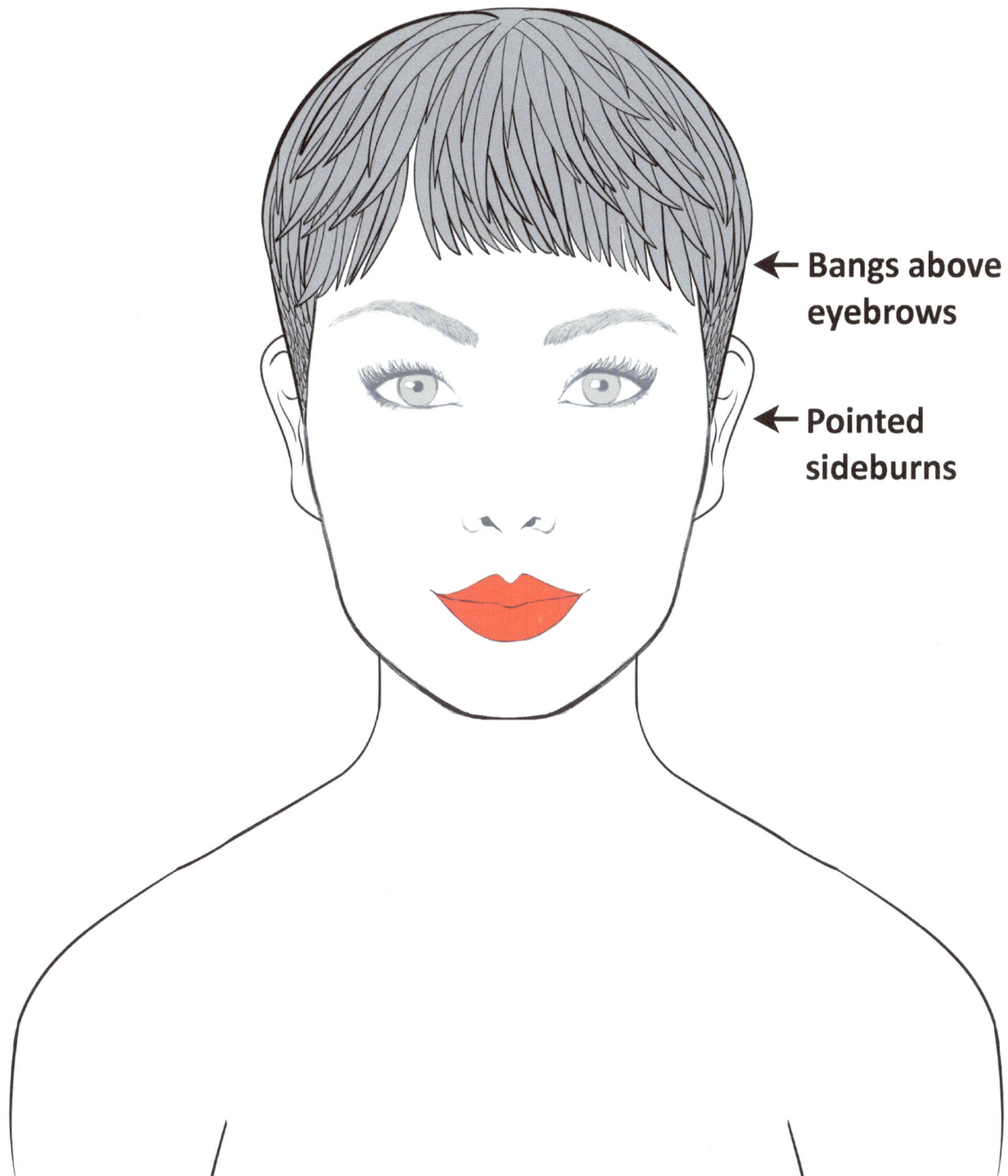

← **Bangs above eyebrows**

← **Pointed sideburns**

SHORT LENGTH - SHORT BANGS

THE PIXIE HAIRCUT

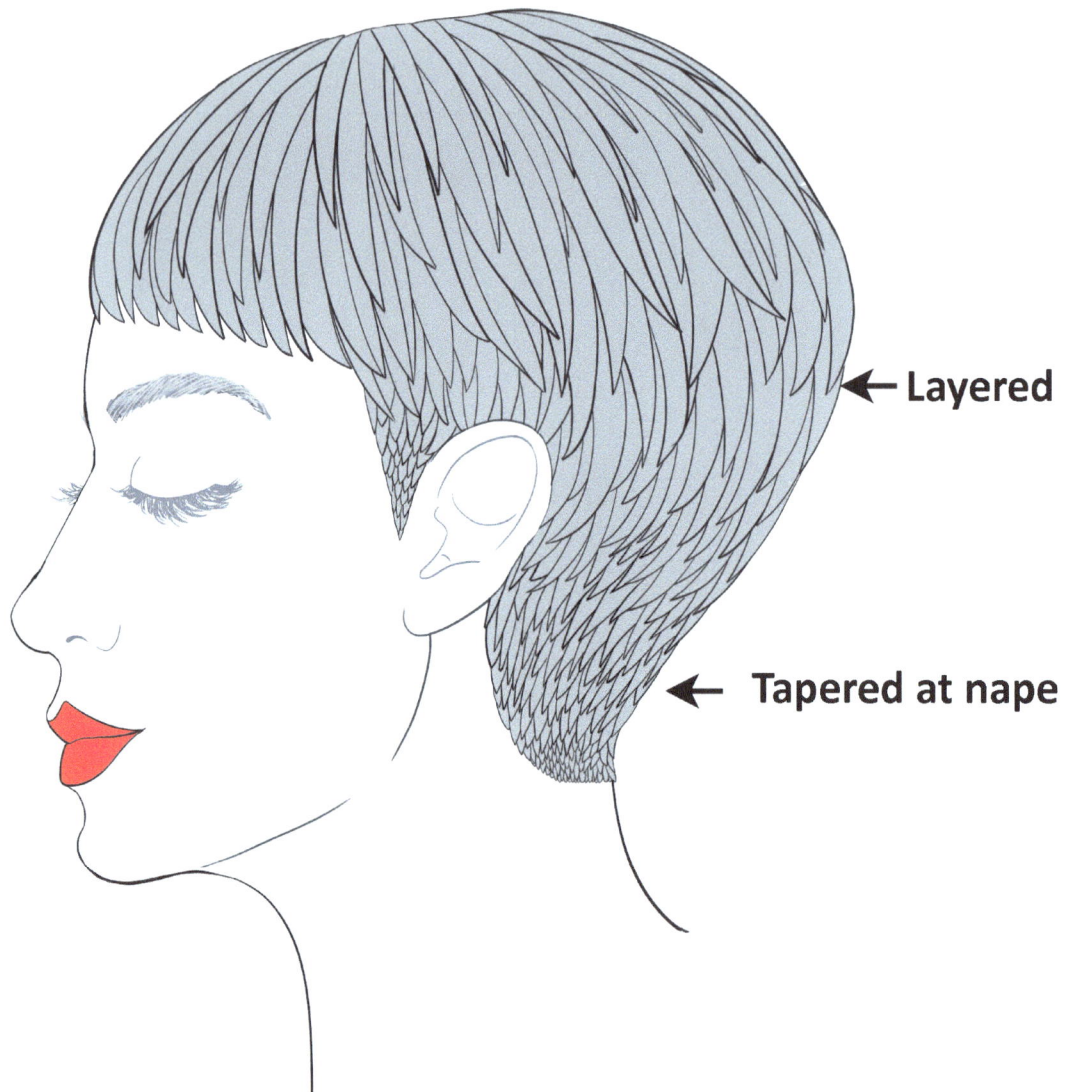

← Layered

← Tapered at nape

SHORT LENGTH - SHORT BANGS

THE PIXIE HAIRCUT

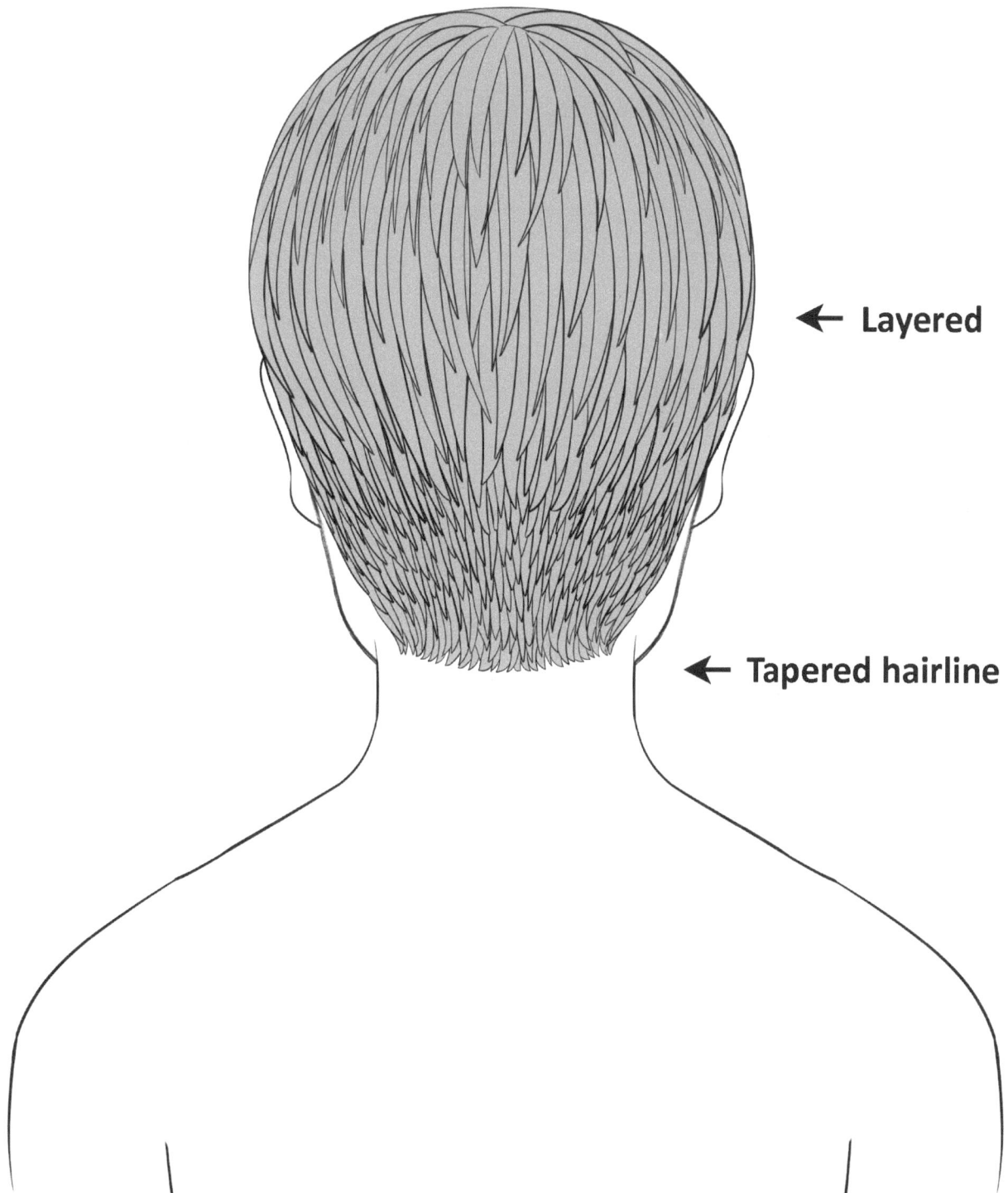

← Layered

← Tapered hairline

SHORT LENGTH - SHORT BANGS

THE PIXIE HAIRCUT

Ear Options

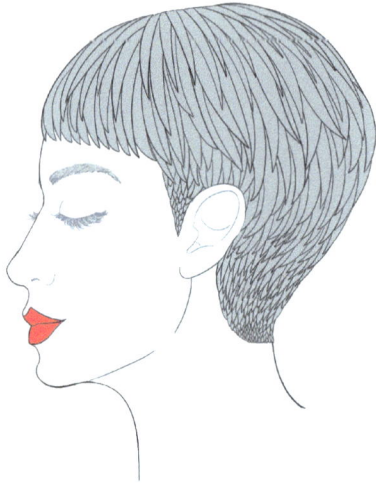

Pointed Sideburns

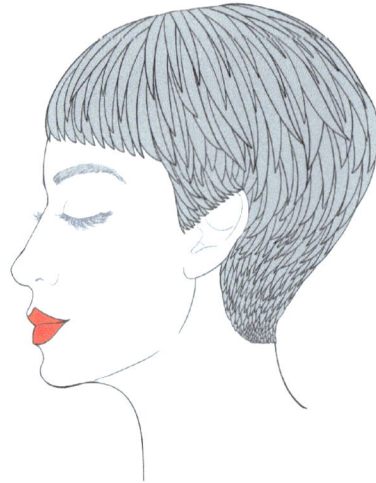

Angled Sideburns

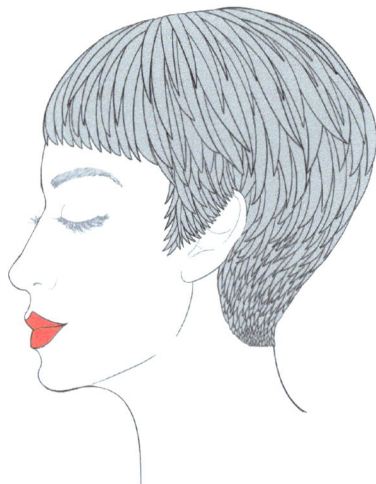

Wispy Sideburns

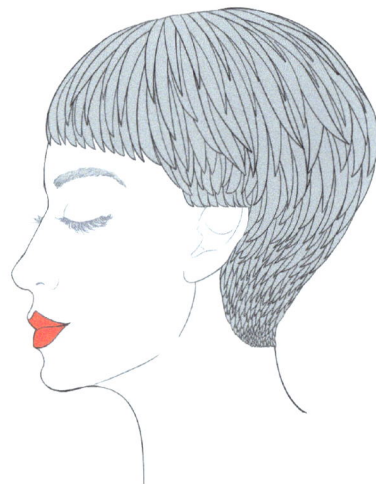

Top of Ear Covered

SHORT LENGTH - SHORT BANGS

THE PIXIE HAIRCUT

Hairline Options

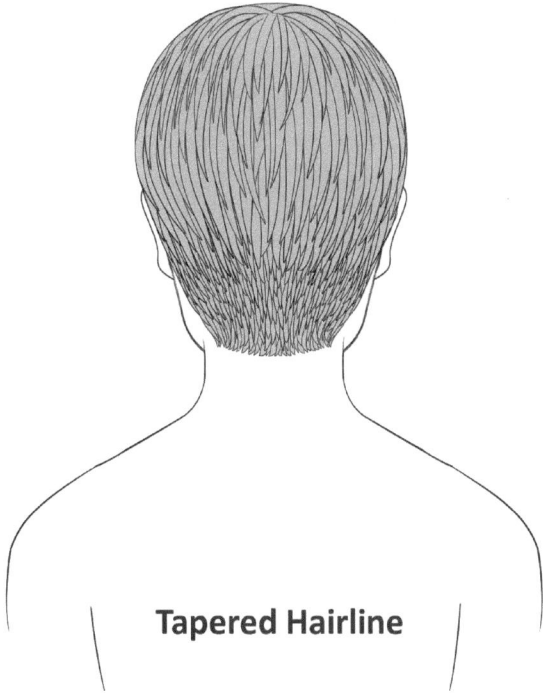

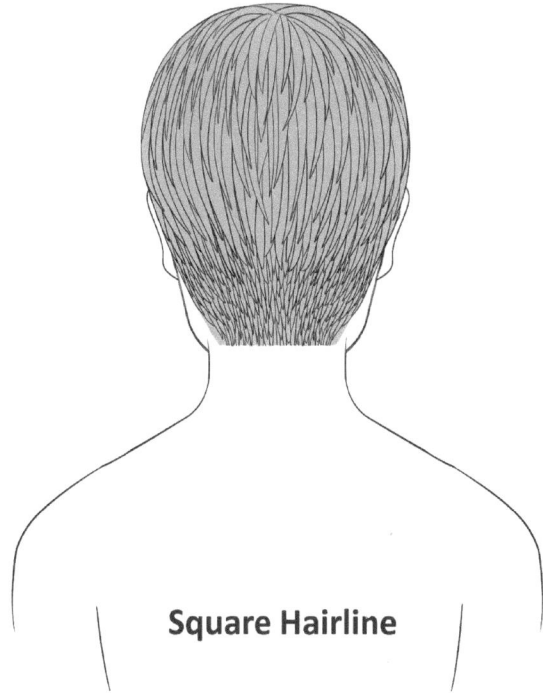

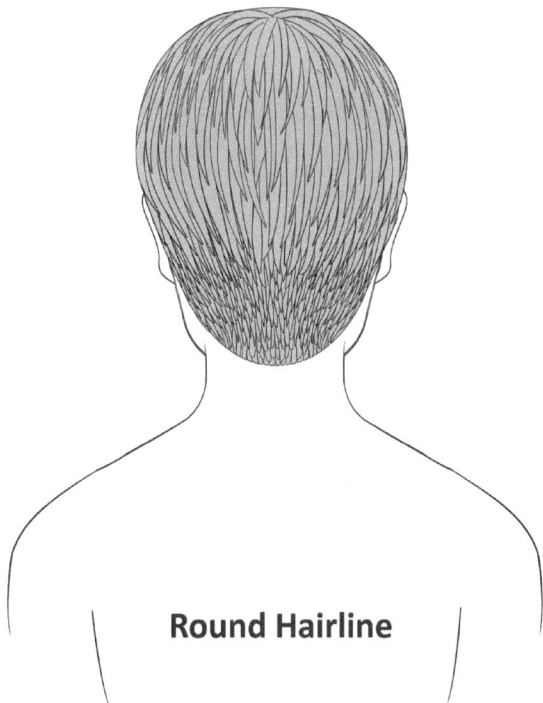

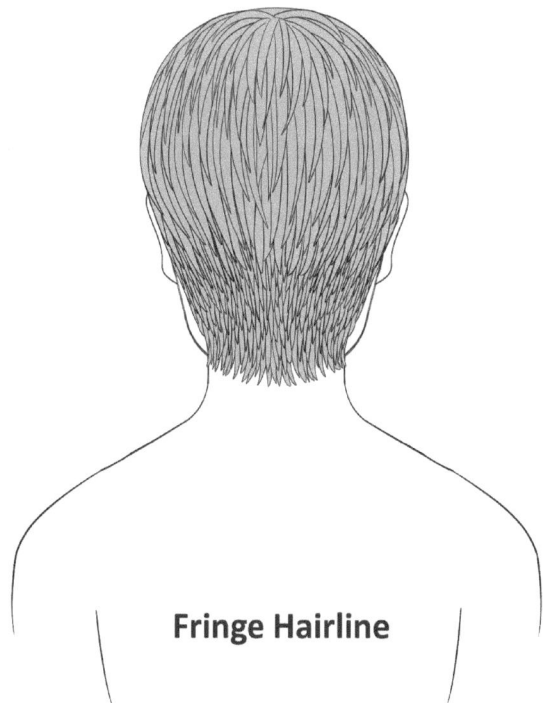

Tapered Hairline

Square Hairline

Round Hairline

Fringe Hairline

SHORT LENGTH - SHORT BANGS

THE PIXIE HAIRCUT

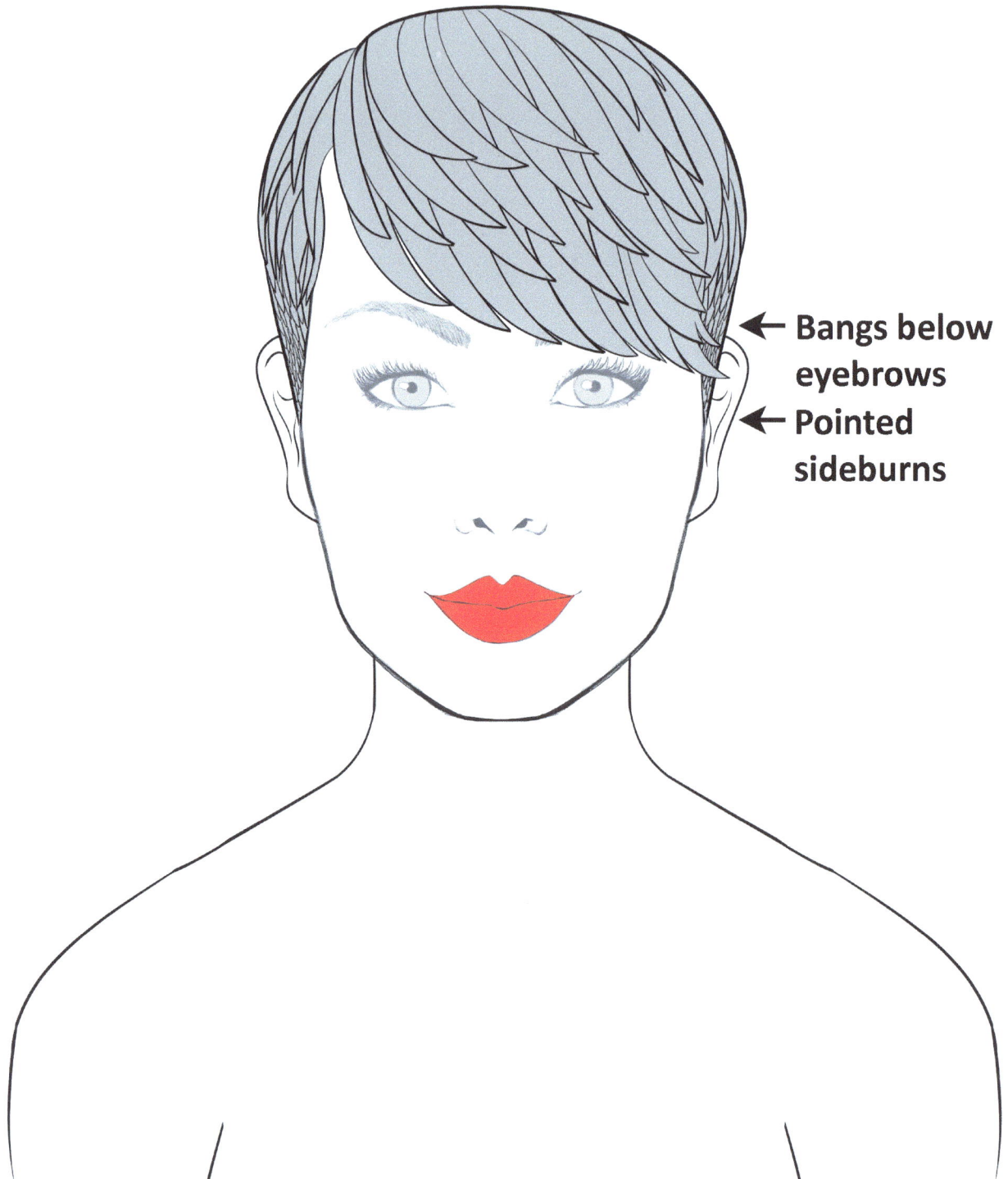

← **Bangs below eyebrows**

← **Pointed sideburns**

SHORT LENGTH - LONG BANGS

THE PIXIE HAIRCUT

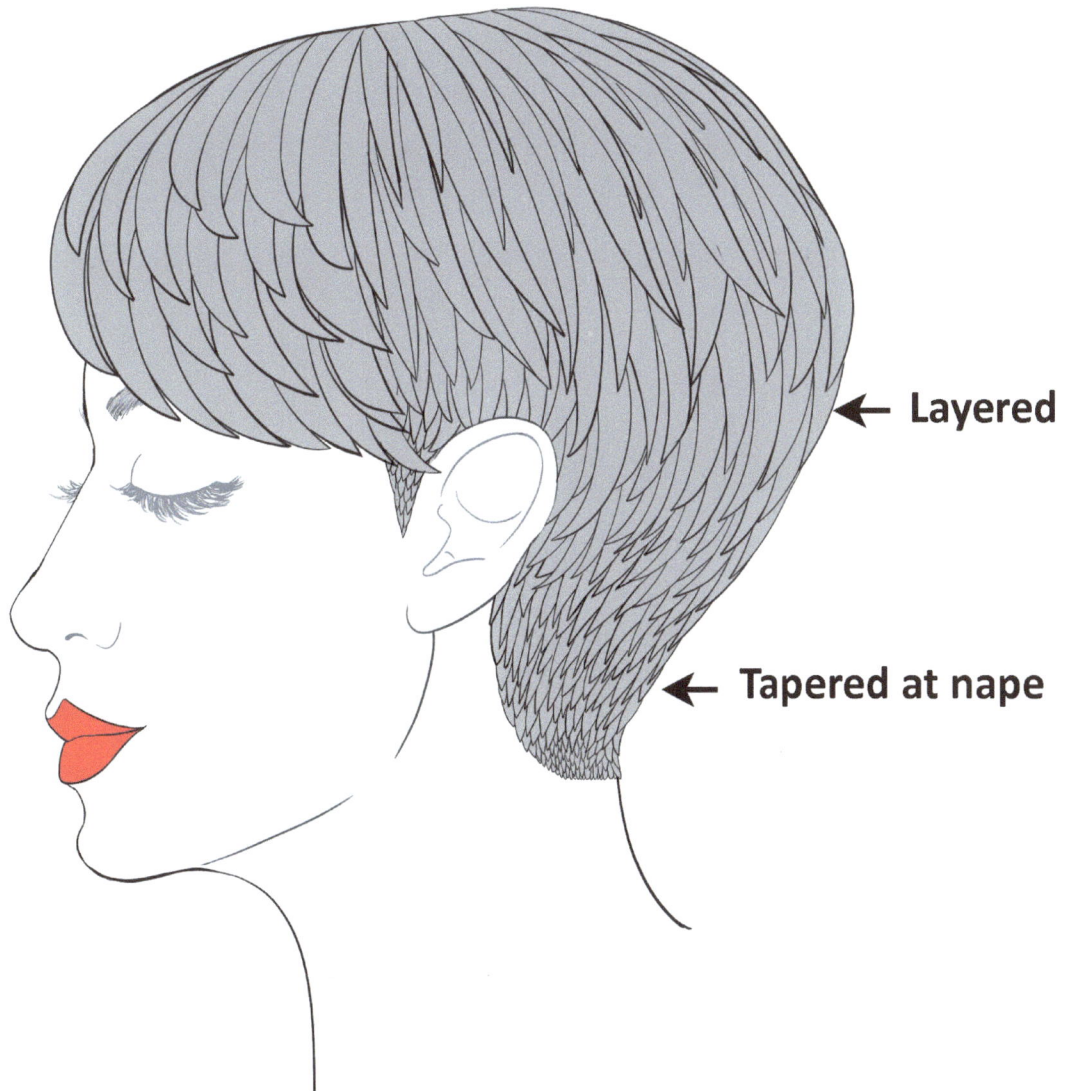

← **Layered**

← **Tapered at nape**

SHORT LENGTH - LONG BANGS

THE PIXIE HAIRCUT

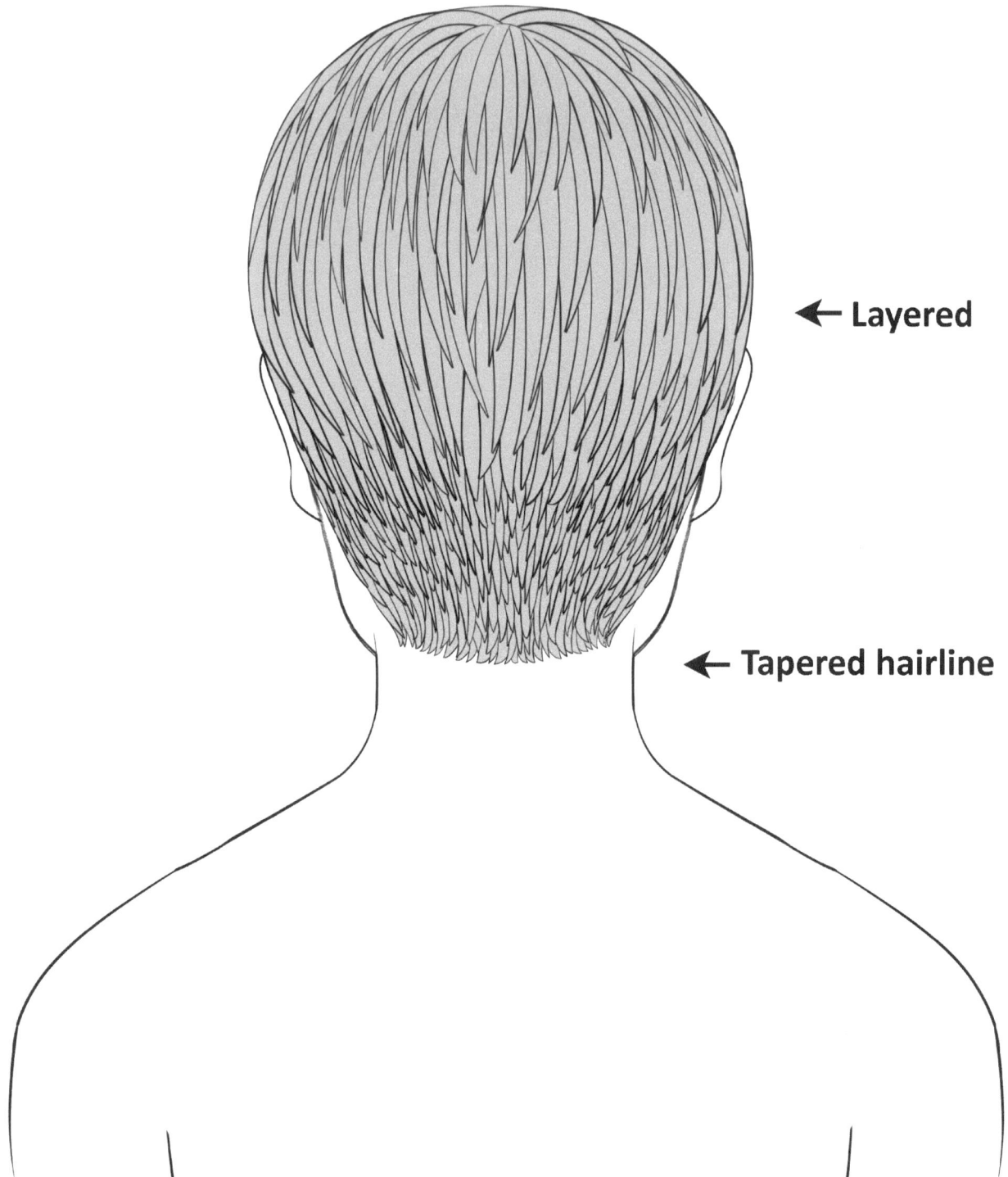

← Layered

← Tapered hairline

SHORT LENGTH - LONG BANGS

THE PIXIE HAIRCUT

Ear Options

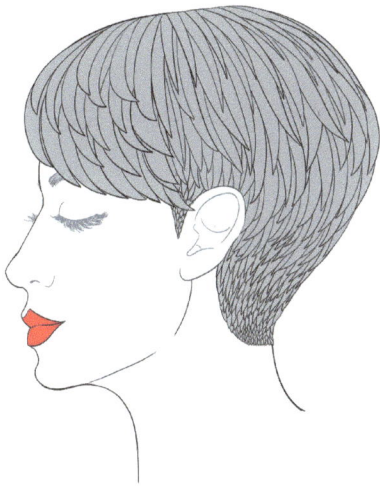

Pointed Sideburns

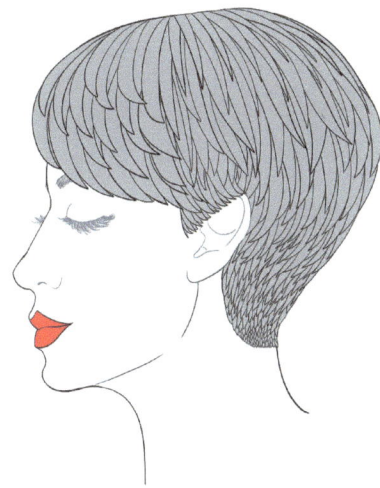

Angled Sideburns

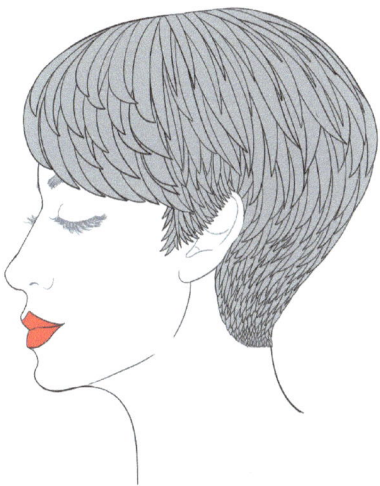

Wispy Sideburns

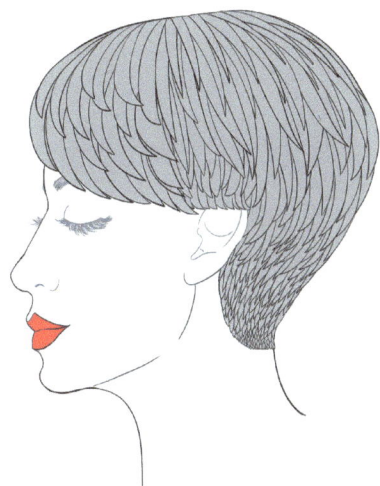

Top of Ear Covered

SHORT LENGTH - LONG BANGS

THE PIXIE HAIRCUT

Hairline Options

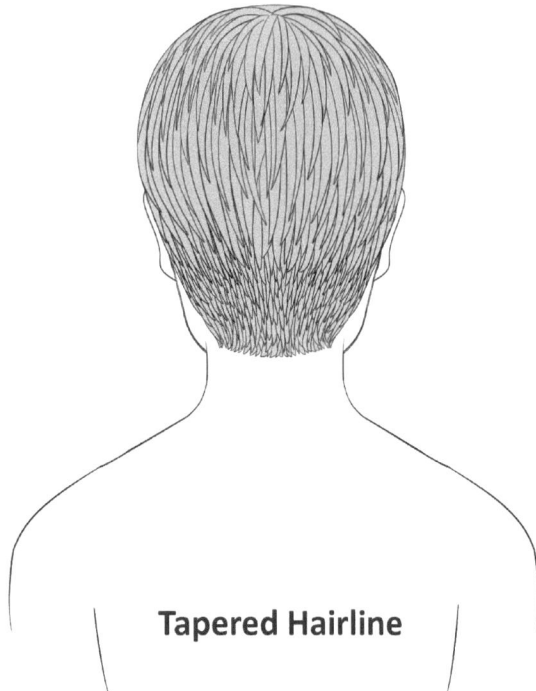

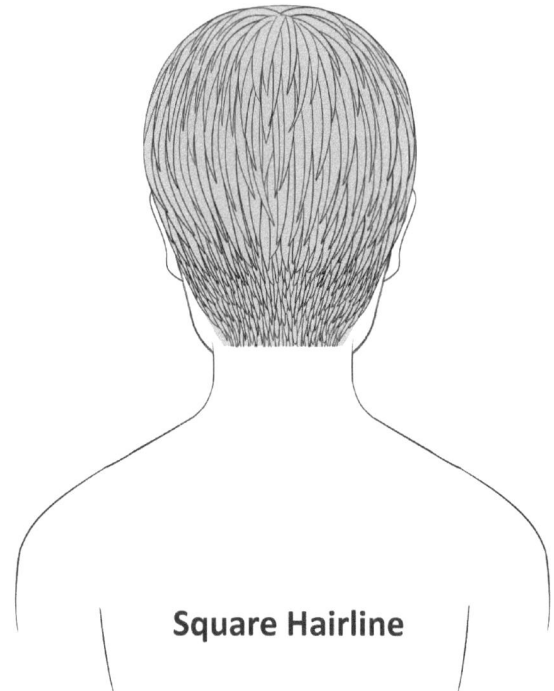

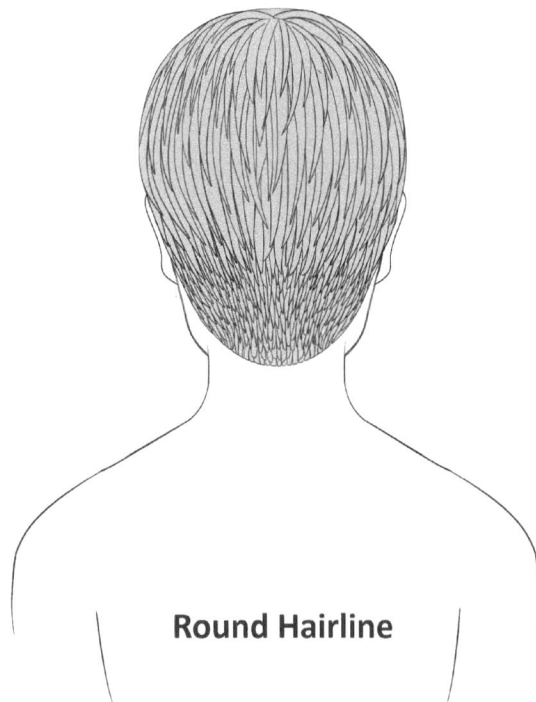

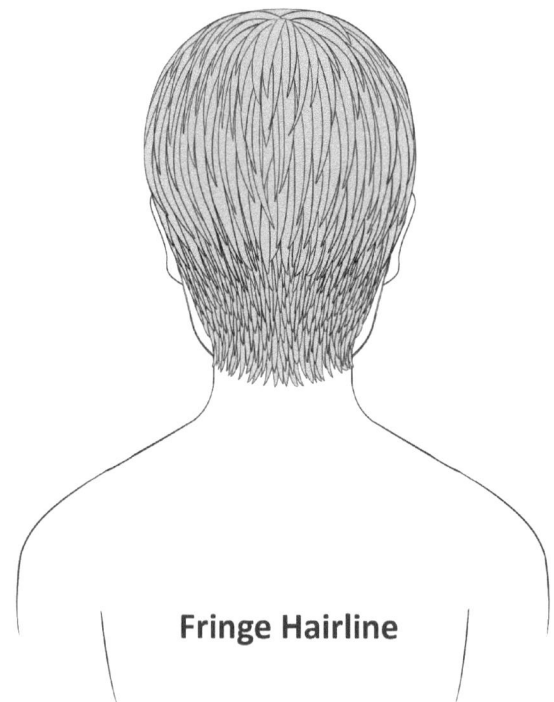

Tapered Hairline

Square Hairline

Round Hairline

Fringe Hairline

SHORT LENGTH - LONG BANGS

THE PIXIE HAIRCUT

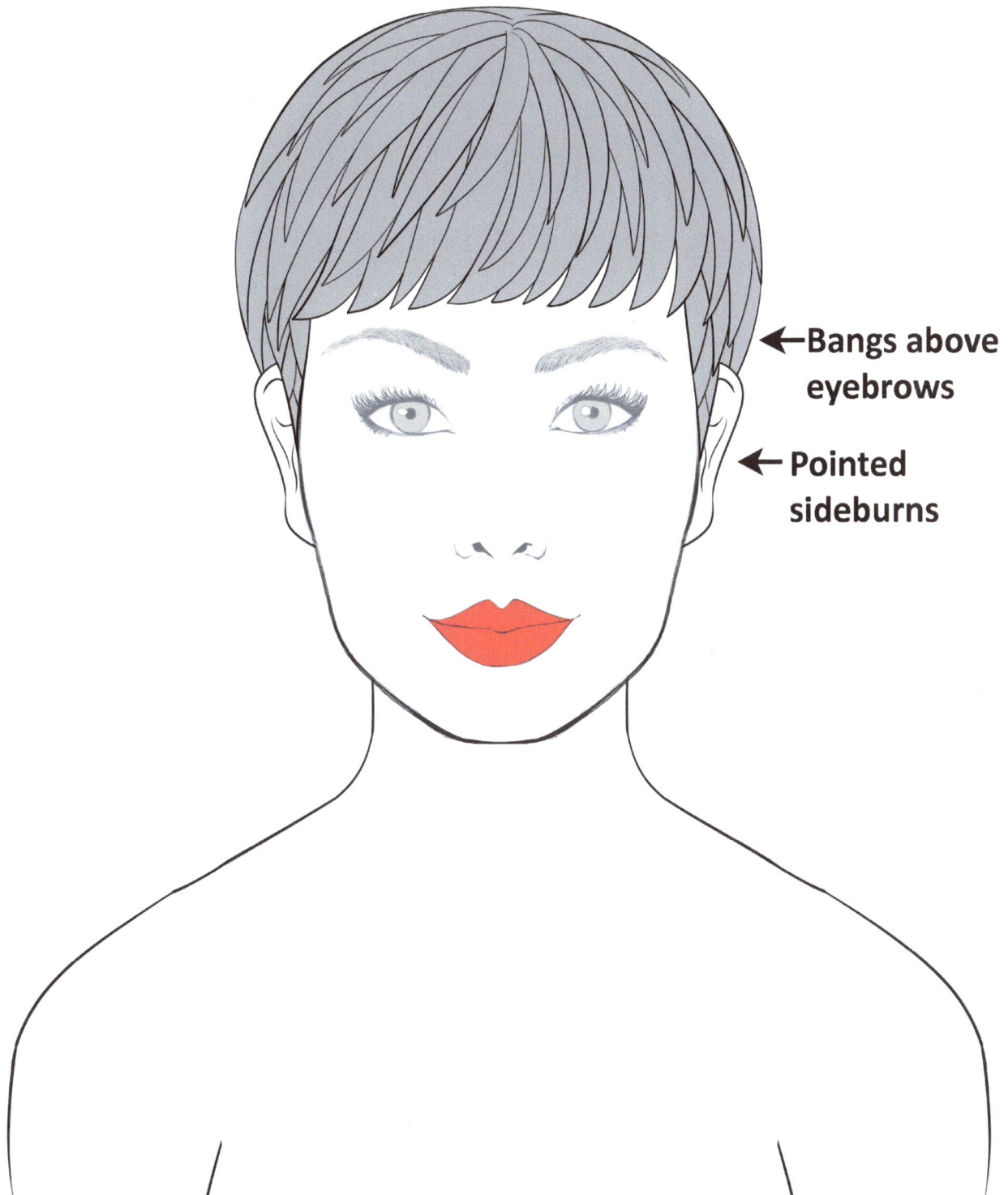

← Bangs above eyebrows

← Pointed sideburns

MEDIUM LENGTH - SHORT BANGS

THE PIXIE HAIRCUT

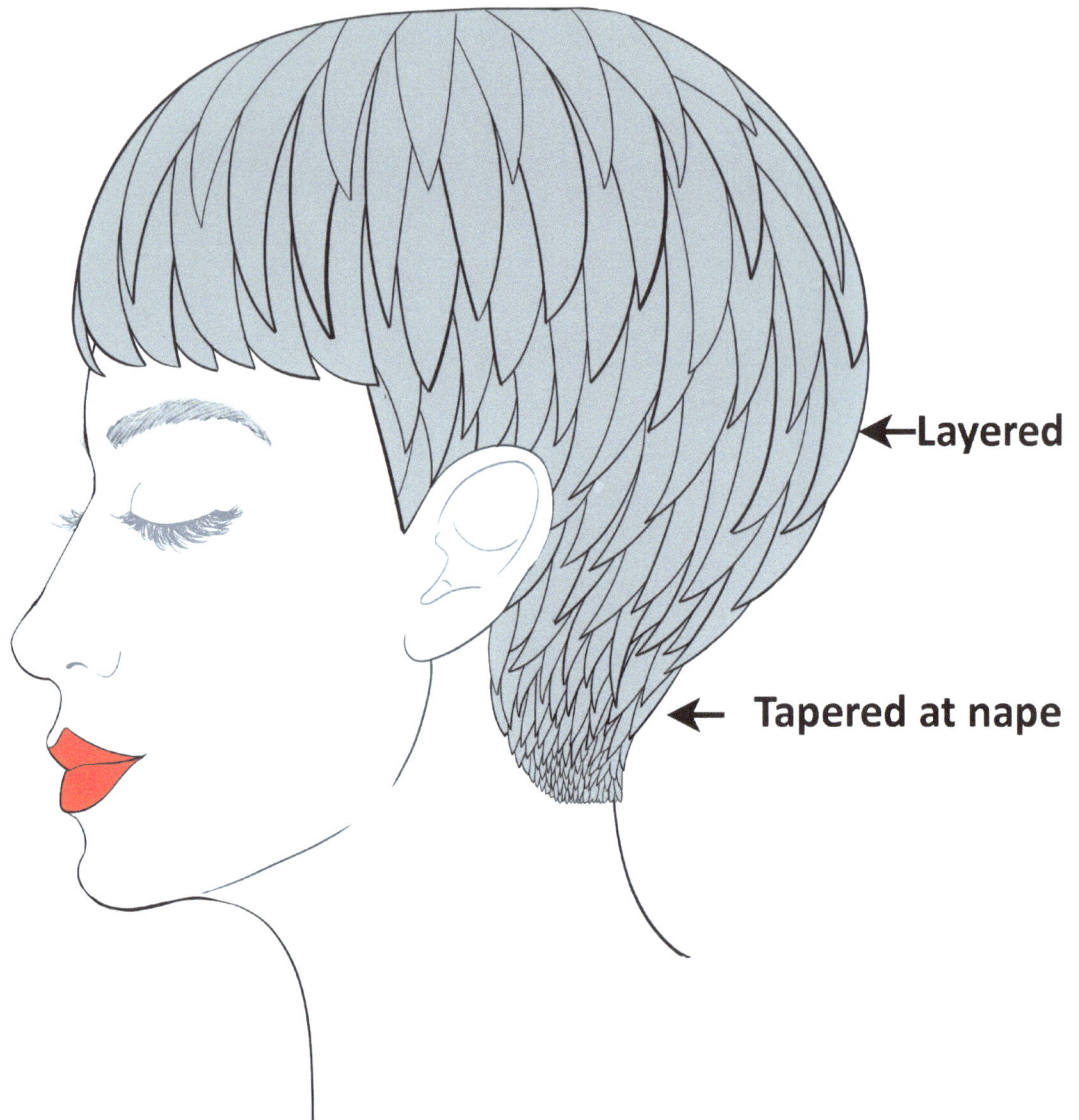

←Layered

← Tapered at nape

MEDIUM LENGTH - SHORT BANGS

THE PIXIE HAIRCUT

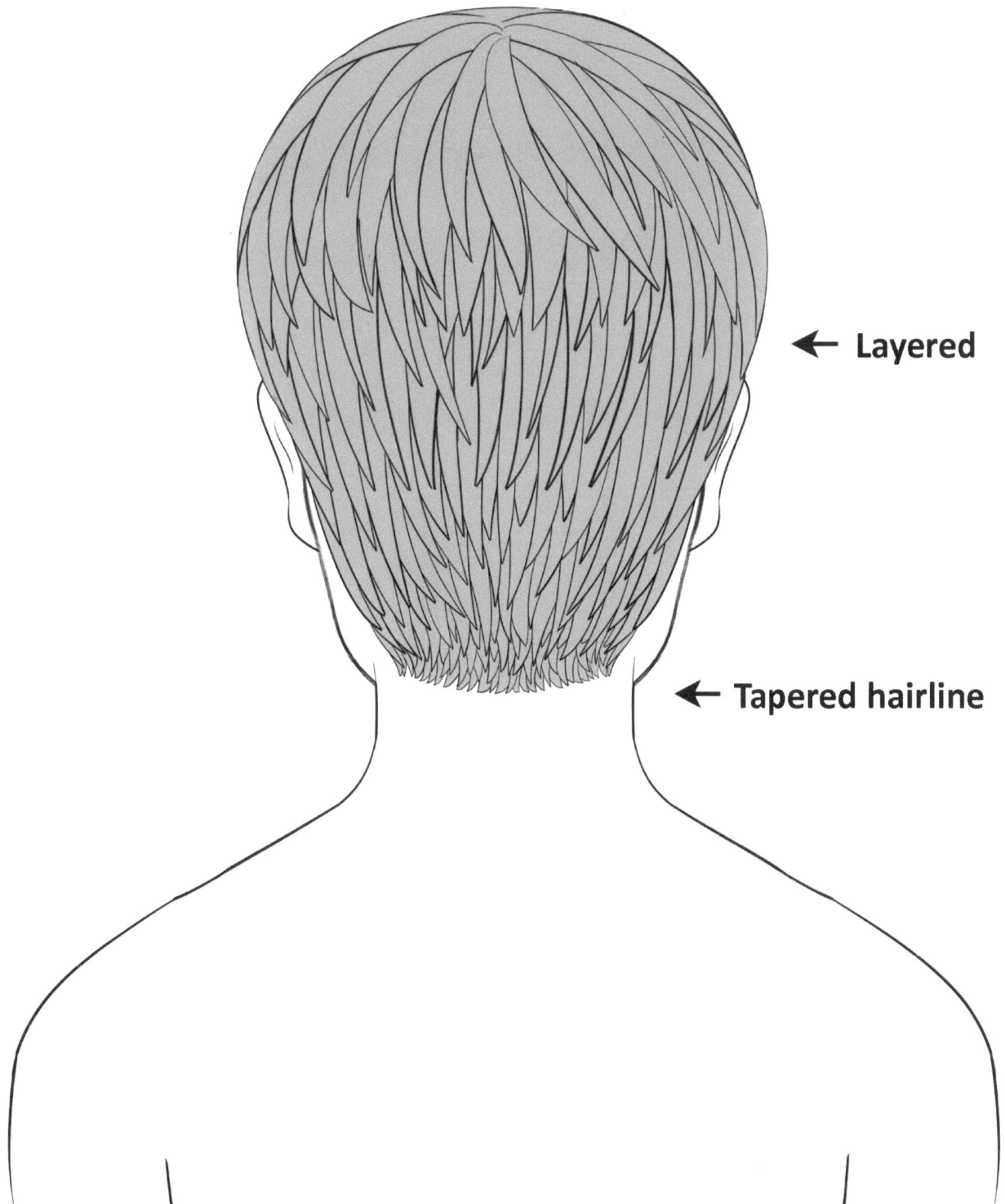

← Layered

← Tapered hairline

MEDIUM LENGTH - SHORT BANGS

THE PIXIE HAIRCUT

Ear Options

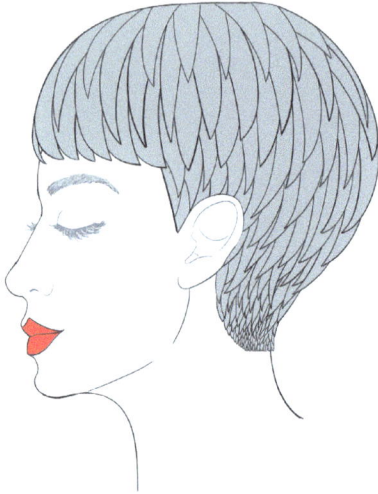

Pointed Sideburns

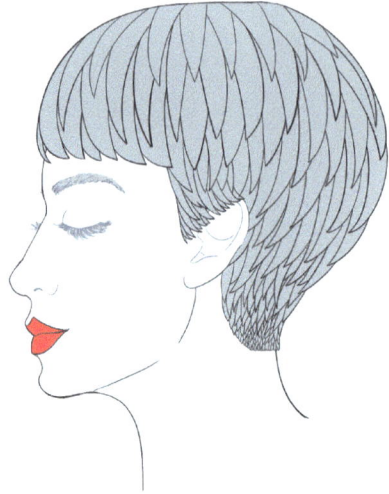

Angled Sideburns

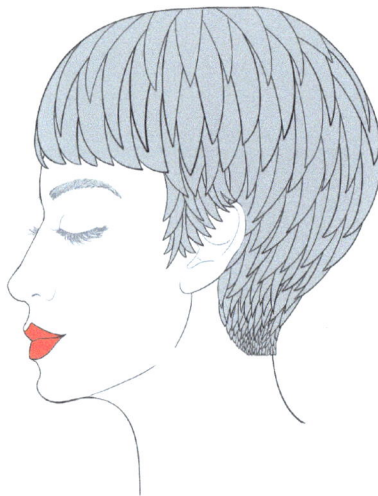

Wispy Sideburns

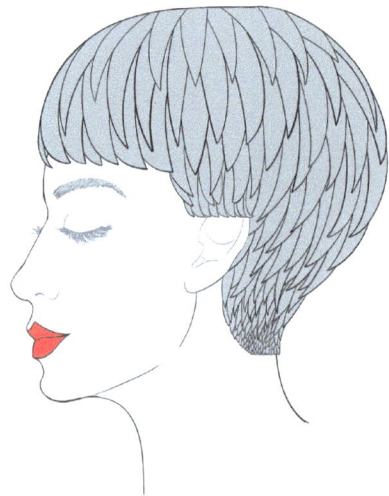

Top of Ear Covered

MEDIUM LENGTH - SHORT BANGS

THE PIXIE HAIRCUT

Hairline Options

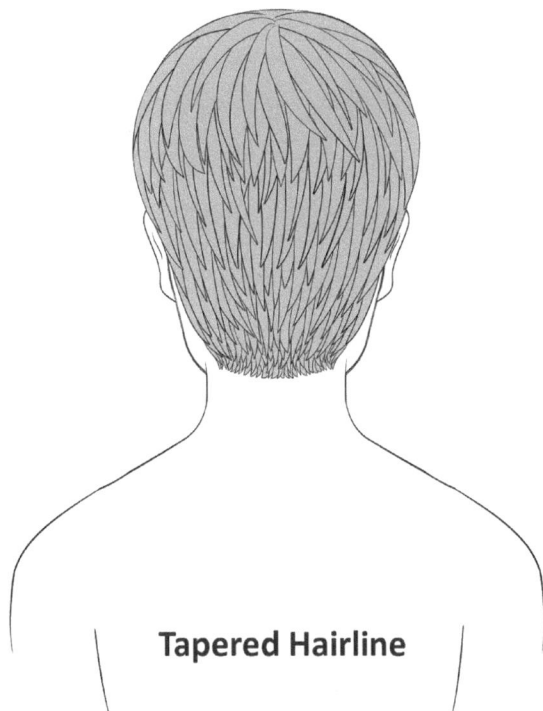

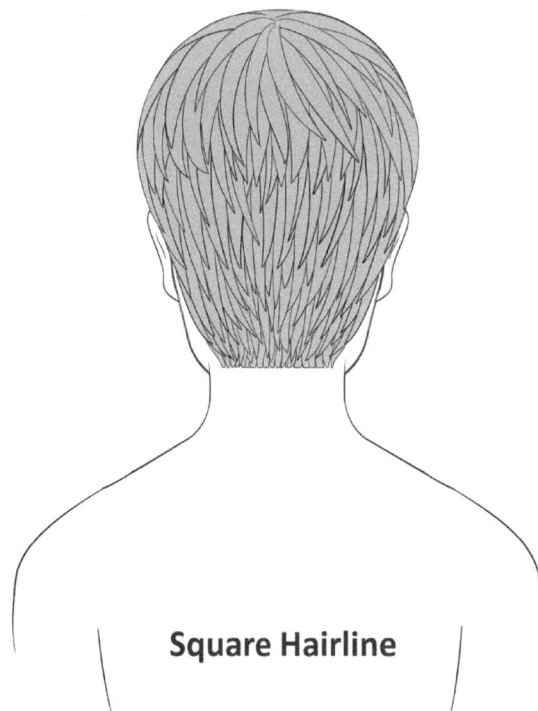

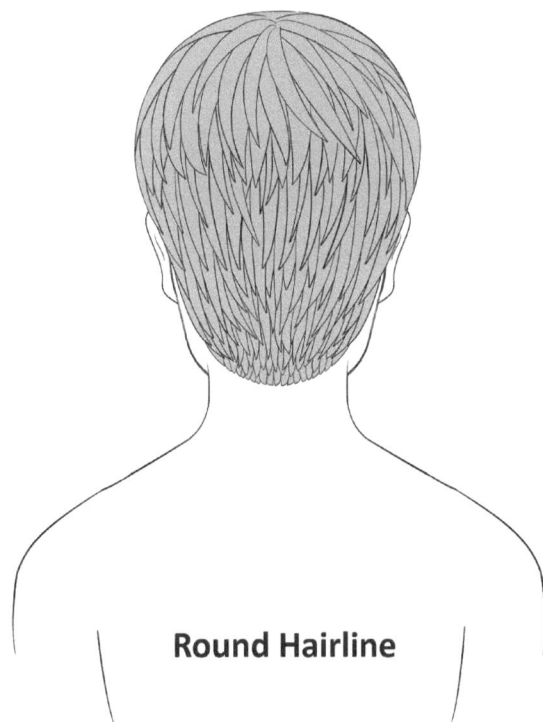

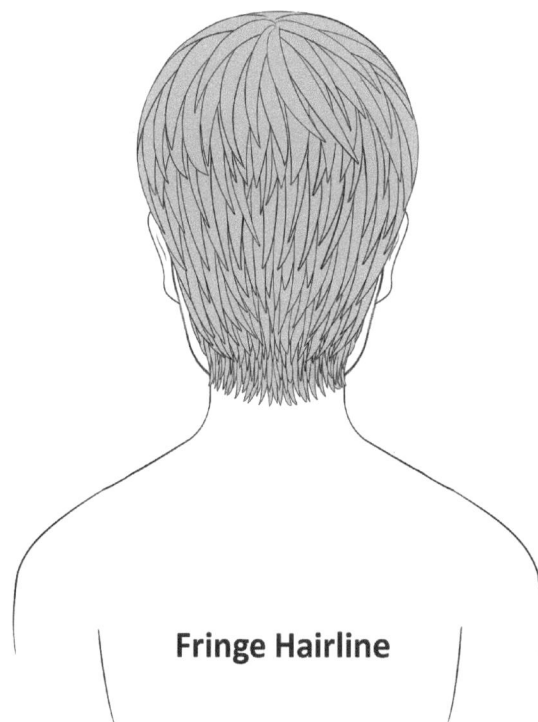

Tapered Hairline

Square Hairline

Round Hairline

Fringe Hairline

MEDIUM LENGTH - SHORT BANGS

THE PIXIE HAIRCUT

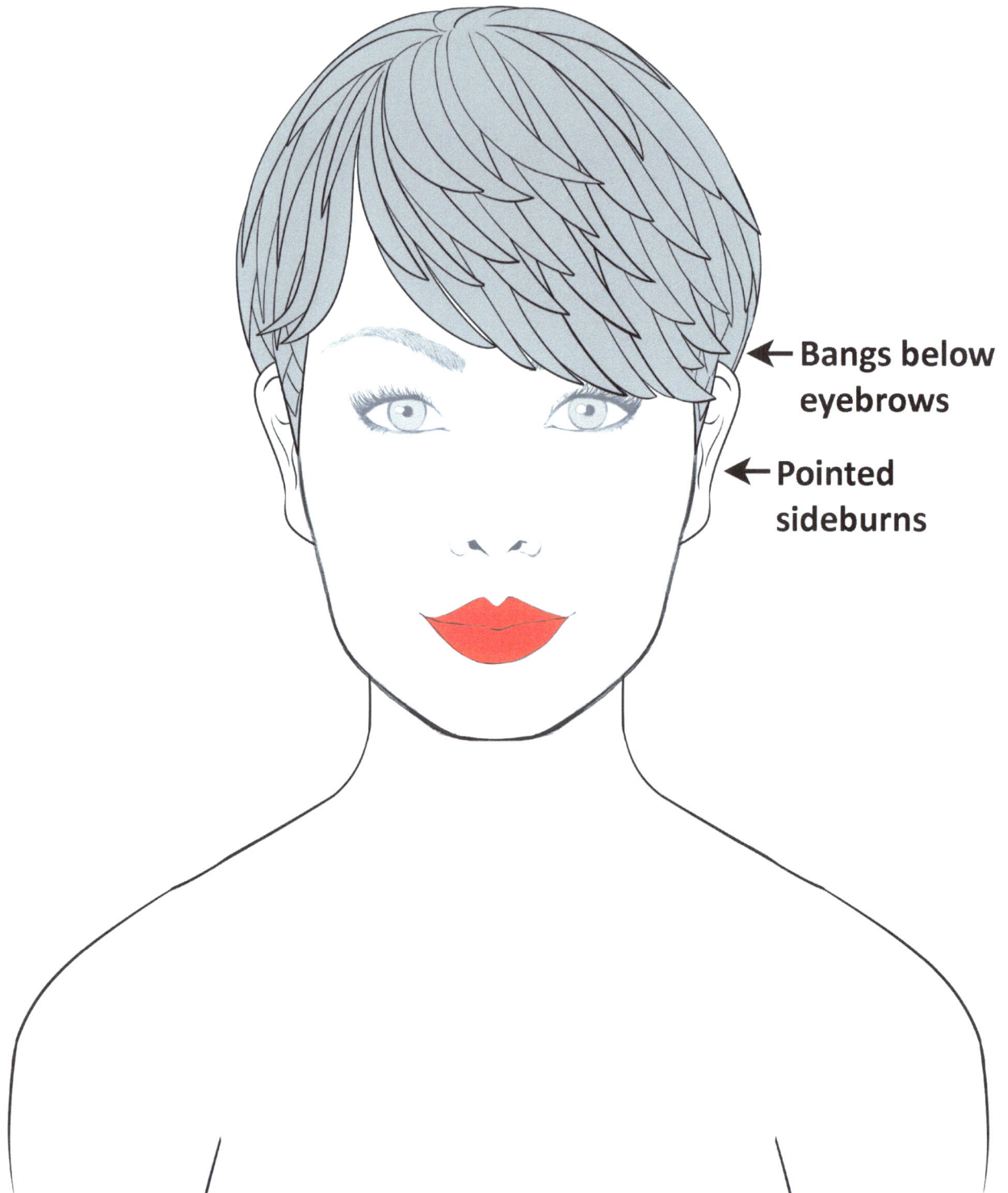

← Bangs below
eyebrows

← Pointed
sideburns

MEDIUM LENGTH - LONG BANGS

THE PIXIE HAIRCUT

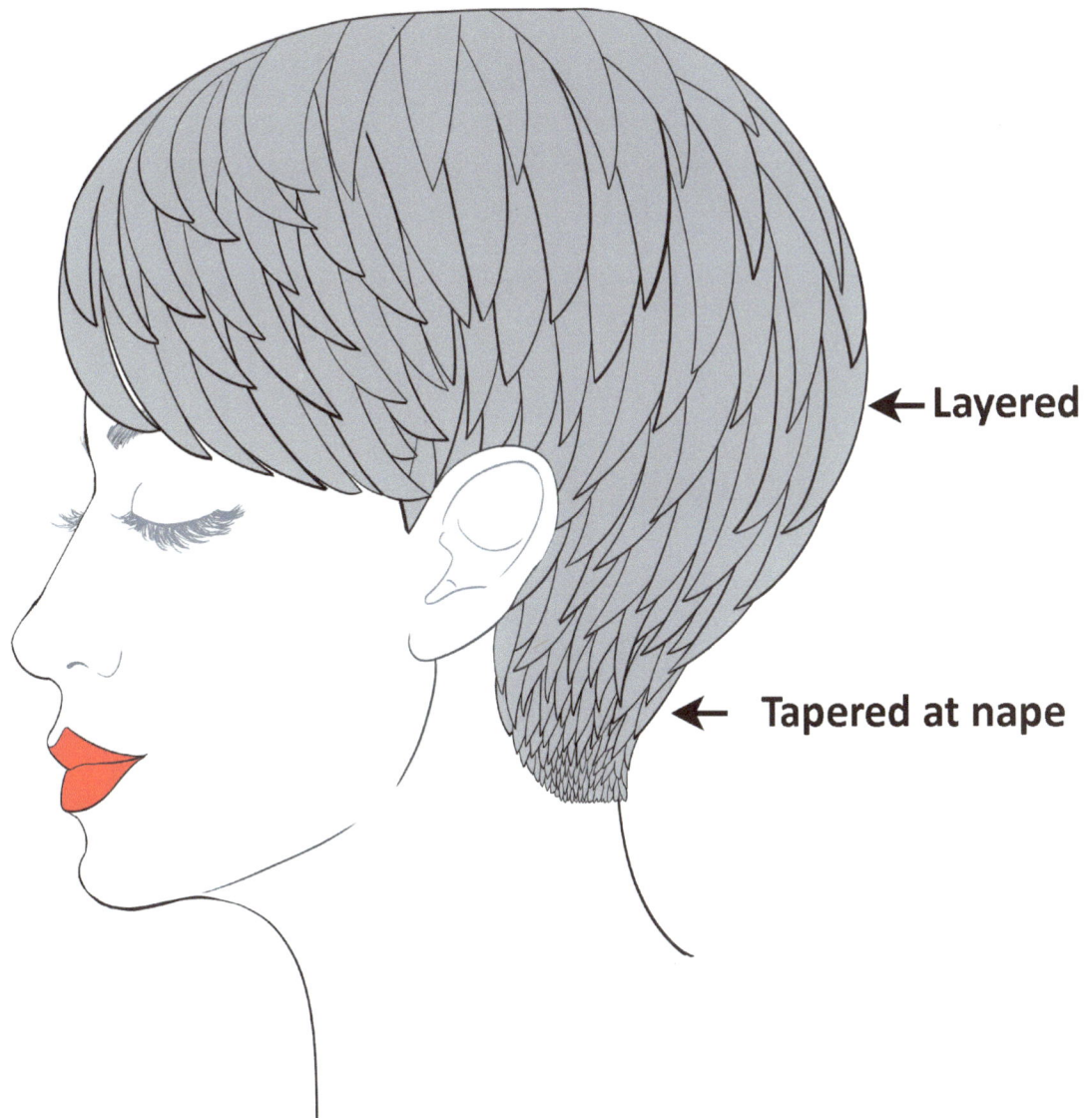

← Layered

← Tapered at nape

MEDIUM LENGTH - LONG BANGS

THE PIXIE HAIRCUT

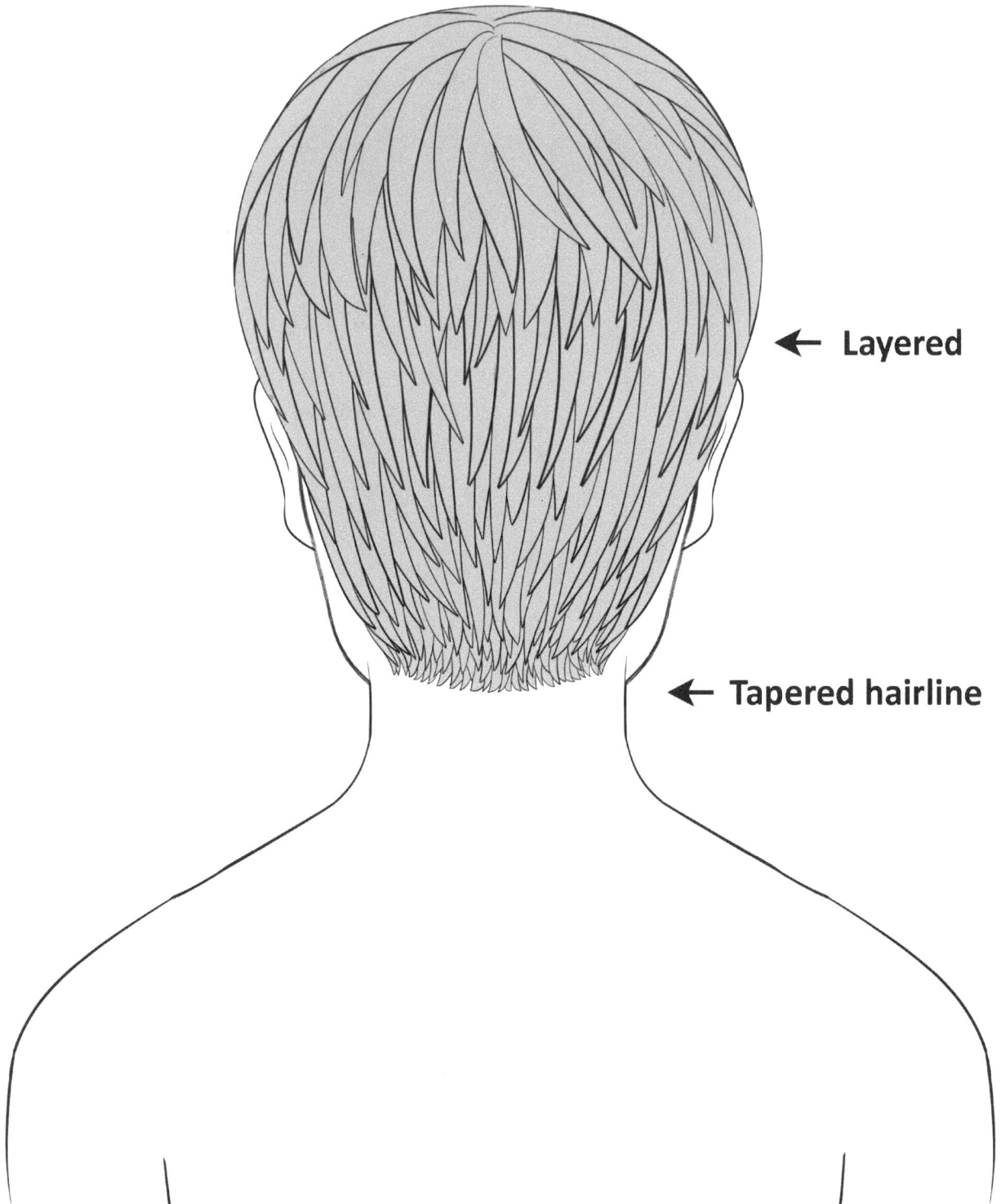

← Layered

← Tapered hairline

MEDIUM LENGTH - LONG BANGS

THE PIXIE HAIRCUT

Ear Options

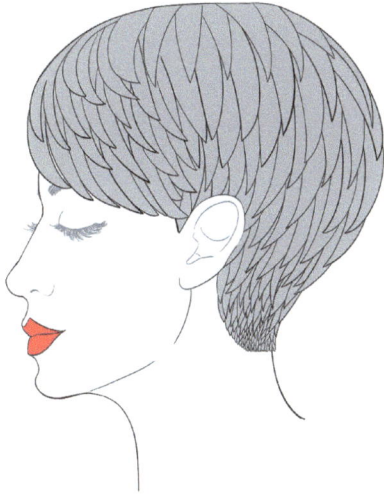

Pointed Sideburns

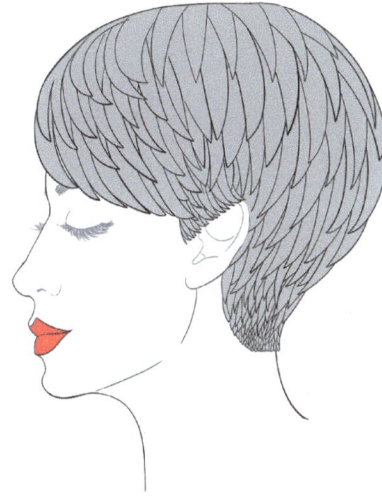

Angled Sideburns

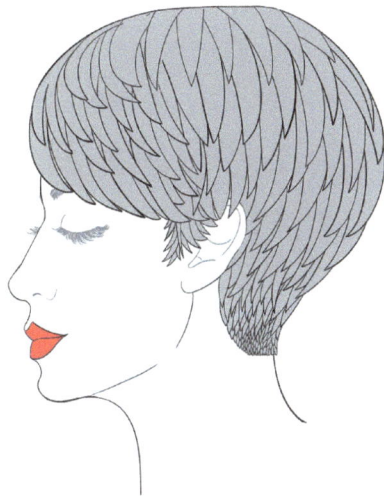

Wispy Sideburns

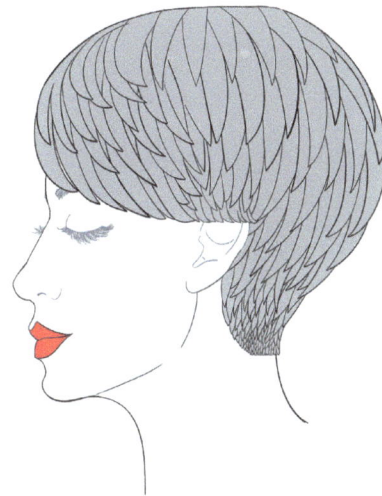

Top of Ear Covered

MEDIUM LENGTH - LONG BANGS

THE PIXIE HAIRCUT

Hairline Options

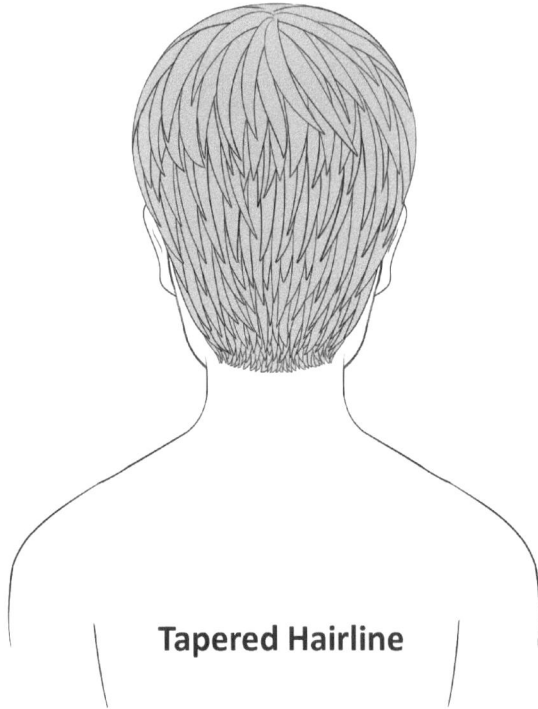

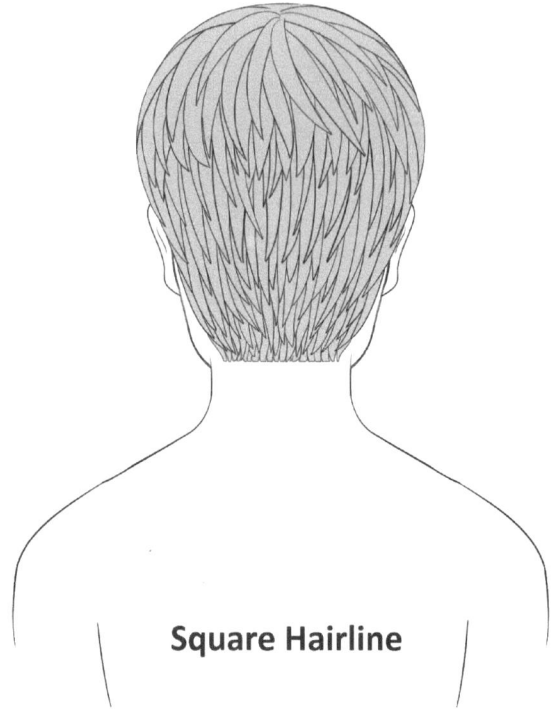

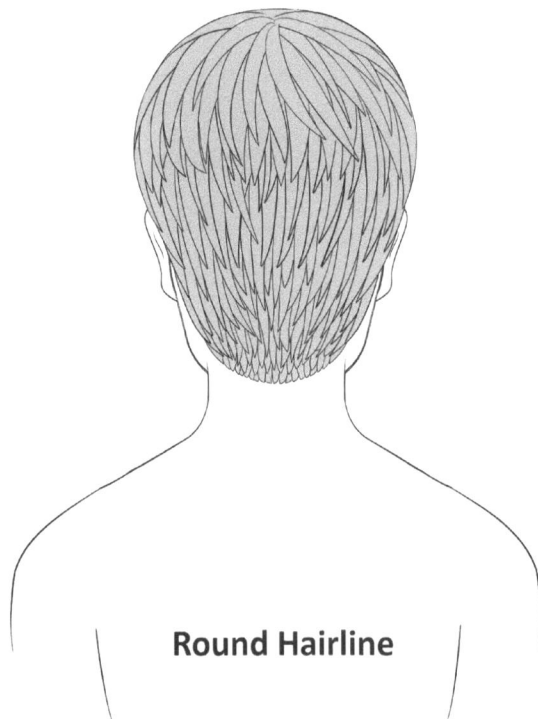

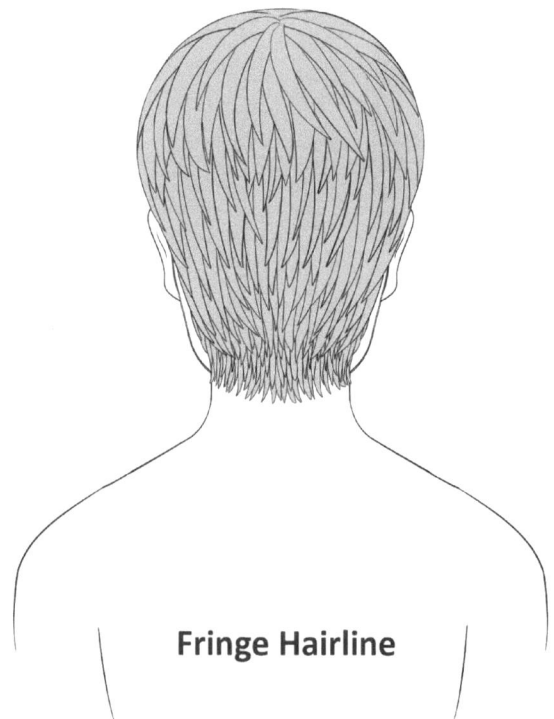

Tapered Hairline

Square Hairline

Round Hairline

Fringe Hairline

MEDIUM LENGTH - LONG BANGS

www.ingramcontent.com/pod-product-compliance
Lightning Source LLC
Chambersburg PA
CBHW061139030426

42335CB00002B/44